The Ultimate Dash Diet Recipes for Soups Lovers

A Guide to Help You Preparing Tasty and Healthy Meals and Enjoy Your Diet

Maya Wilson

© **Copyright 2021 - All rights reserved.**

The content contained within this book may not be reproduced, duplicated or transmitted without direct written permission from the author or the publisher.

Under no circumstances will any blame or legal responsibility be held against the publisher, or author, for any damages, reparation, or monetary loss due to the information contained within this book. Either directly or indirectly.

Legal Notice:

This book is copyright protected. This book is only for personal use. You cannot amend, distribute, sell, use, quote or paraphrase any part, or the content within this book, without the consent of the author or publisher.

Disclaimer Notice:

Please note the information contained within this document is for educational and entertainment purposes only. All effort has been executed to present accurate, up to date, and reliable, complete information. No warranties of any kind are declared or implied. Readers acknowledge that the author is not engaging in the rendering of legal, financial, medical or professional advice. The content within this book has been derived from various sources. Please consult a licensed professional before attempting any techniques outlined in this book.

By reading this document, the reader agrees that under no circumstances is the author responsible for any losses, direct or indirect, which are incurred as a result of the use of information contained within this document, including, but not limited to, — errors, omissions, or inaccuracies.

Table of contents

- Chicken, Lentil, and Spinach Soup 5
- Roasted Tomato Basil Soup 9
- Roasted Red Pepper and Tomato Soup 11
- Mushroom & Broccoli Soup 15
- Creamy Cauliflower Pakora Soup 17
- Garden Vegetable and Herb Soup 20
- Super-easy Chicken Noodle Soup 23
- Hearty Ginger Soup 27
- Tasty Tofu and Mushroom Soup 30
- Ingenious Eggplant Soup 32
- Loving Cauliflower Soup 35
- Simple Garlic and Lemon Soup 38
- Healthy Cucumber Soup 41
- Mushroom Cream Soup 43
- Curious Roasted Garlic Soup 45
- Amazing Roasted Carrot Soup 48
- Simple Pumpkin Soup 50
- Coconut Avocado Soup 52
- Coconut Arugula Soup 54
- Awesome Cabbage Soup 57
- Ginger Zucchini Avocado Soup 59
- Greek Lemon and Chicken Soup 62
- Morning Peach 65
- Garlic and Pumpkin Soup 67
- Butternut and Garlic Soup 70
- Minty Avocado Soup 72
- Celery, Cucumber and Zucchini Soup 75
- Rosemary and Thyme Cucumber Soup 77
- Guacamole Soup 80
- Cucumber and Zucchini Soup 82
- Crockpot Pumpkin Soup 84
- Tomato Soup 87
- Pumpkin, Coconut and Sage Soup 90
- Sweet Potato and Leek Soup 92
- The Kale and Spinach Soup 94
- Japanese Onion Soup 97
- Amazing Broccoli and Cauliflower Soup 99
- Amazing Zucchini Soup 102

PORTUGUESE KALE AND SAUSAGE SOUP 104
DAZZLING PIZZA SOUP 107

Chicken, Lentil, and Spinach Soup

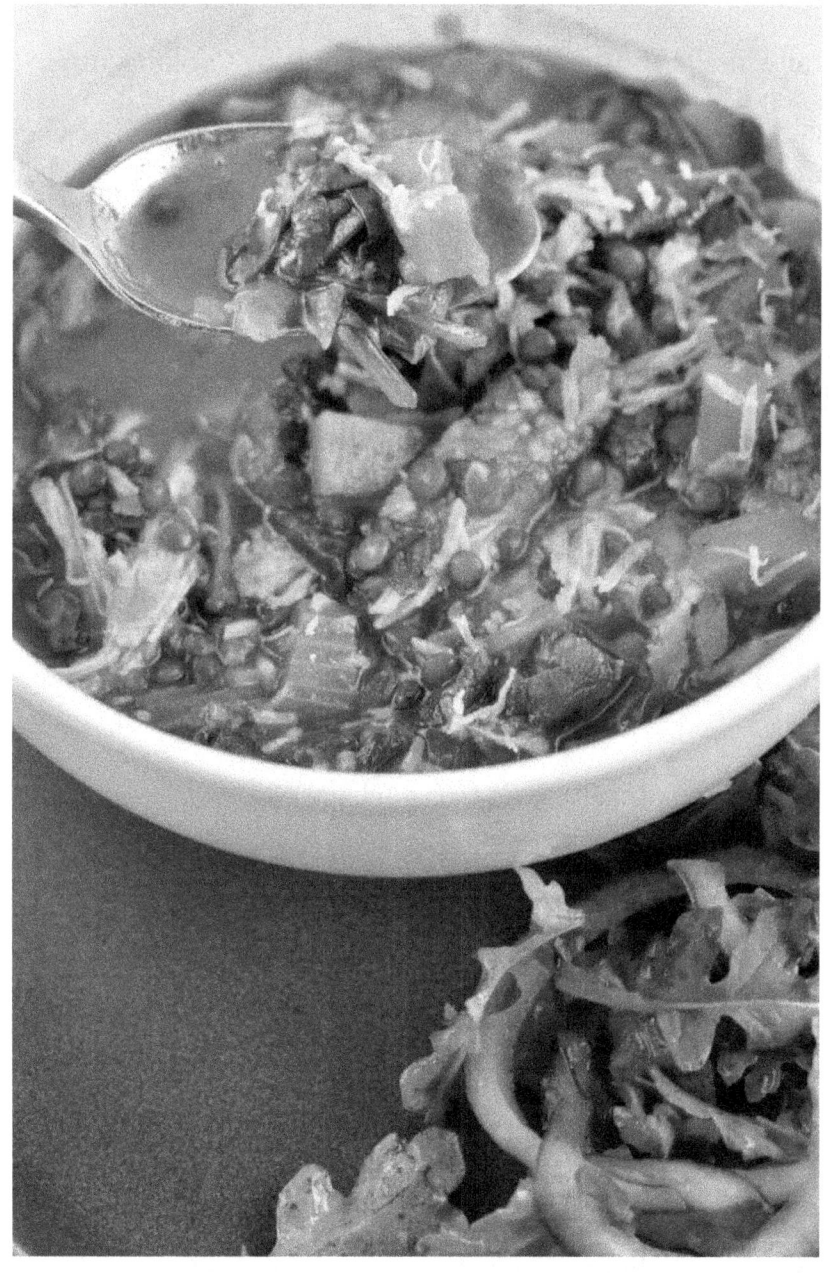

SmartPoints value: Green plan - 1SP, Blue plan - 1SP, Purple plan - 1SP

Total Time: 1hr 10min, Prep time: 10 min, Cooking time: 1hr, Serves: 6

Nutritional value: Calories – 254, Carbs – 27g, Fat – 4.8g, Protein – 26g

As I said earlier, soups and stews are great for me during fall and winter, but this chicken, lentil, and spinach could also serve as spring meals. Though not as rich and heavy as other soups, it is quite substantial.

Ingredients

- Chicken breast - 1 lb

- French dried (green lentils) - 1 cup

- Fresh spinach - One 6 oz package

- Finely chopped onion (1 piece)

- Carrots (chopped) - 2 pieces

- Stalk of celery (chopped) - 2 pieces

- Garlic (chopped) - 6 cloves

- Olive oil (1 tbsp)

- Tomato paste - 2 tbsp

- Paprika - 1 tsp

- Chicken broth or water - 6 cups (fat-free)

- Fresh lemon juice – Half a cup

- Add salt and pepper to taste

Instructions

1. Use medium heat to heat olive oil in a large pot or Dutch oven

2. Put carrots, celery, onions, and garlic and cook till about minutes when vegetables begin to soften
3. Coat the vegetables with the tomato paste and cover till about 2-3 minutes when the paste begins to darken.
4. Stir lentils, paprika, salt, and pepper in the broth or water and bring to a boil and add in the chicken, then cook for about 5 minutes.

5. Cover and cook for about 35 – 45 minutes on medium-low heat until chicken cooks and lentil are tender but not mushy. Make sure the soup is not bubbling or boiling much as you stir periodically.

6. Shred the chicken breasts using two forks. Stir in spinach and lemon juice and cook for about 2 minutes until the spinach wilts. Turn off the heat and add additional salt and pepper to taste.

7. To enjoy the chicken stew and leave it in mind as your best, do not overcook the lentils. Keep an eye on it and make sure they are tender but firm.

Roasted Tomato Basil Soup

SmartPoints value: Green plan - 4SP, Blue plan - 4SP, Purple plan - 4SP

Total Time: 1hr 20min, Prep time: 10 min, Cooking time: 1hr 10mins,

Serves: 4

Nutritional value: Calories – 238, Carbs – 26.1g, Fat – 3g, Protein – 5g

Most tomato soups are creamy but unfortunately has lots of fat, but this roasted tomato basil soup makes the difference. You might just say goodbye to canned tomato soup after enjoying the fresh flavors of roasted tomato basil soup.

Ingredients

- Plum tomatoes (halved) - 2 lbs

- Plum tomatoes in their juice - One 14 oz can

- Olive oil - 1 tbsp

- Onion (diced) - 1 large

- Minced garlic (4 cloves)

- Butter (2 tbsp)

- Red pepper flakes (crushed) - 1/8 tsp

- Vegetable stock - 3 cups

- Basil (fresh) - 2 cups

- Oregano (dried) - 1 tsp

- Salt and pepper as desired

Instructions

1. Line a rimmed baking sheet with parchment paper on a 400-degree preheated oven. Before placing them on the baking sheet, toss the tomatoes and garlic cloves with olive oil. Then roast for about 35-45 minutes or until tomatoes are charred.

2. Using medium heat, heat the butter in a stockpot or Dutch, then add onions and red pepper flakes. Sauté until the onion starts to brown.

3. In the canned tomato, stir the basil, oregano, and stock or water. Then, add in the oven-roasted tomatoes and garlic, including any juices on the baking sheet. Boil and simmer uncovered for about 25-30, then stir regularly.
4. Until you reach the desired consistency, process the soup using an immersion blender.
5. Add salt and pepper to taste.

Roasted Red Pepper and Tomato Soup

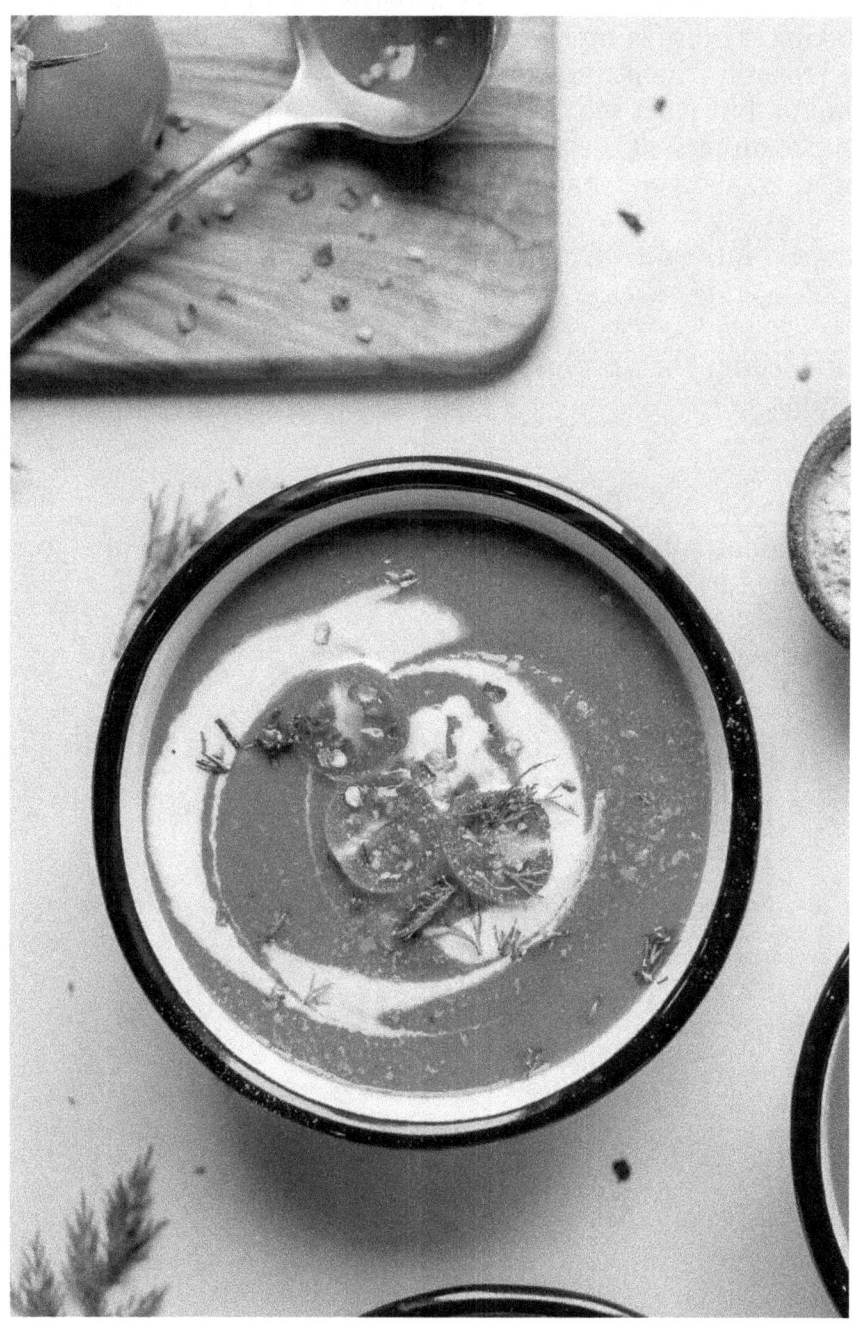

Since my favorite lunch is grilled cheese sandwiches, I had to, of course, make tomato soup as a perfect match, so I thought of making it more sumptuous by adding tomatoes and red pepper and roasting them altogether. It might not be as quick as a canned tomato, but trust me, it's worth every single minute. While the soup simmers, it's easy to put the grilled cheese sandwiches together, and you'll have your desired meal.

SmartPoints value: Green plan - 1SP, Blue plan - 1SP, Purple plan - 1SP

Total Time: 1hr 20min, Prep time: 10 min, Cooking time: 1hr 10mins,

Serves: 6

Nutritional value: Calories – 107, Carbs – 19.4g, Fat – 0.4g, Protein – 4g

Ingredients

- Plum tomatoes - 10 pieces

- Bell peppers (red) - 3 pieces

- Onion - 1 small

- Olive oil - 1 tbsp

- Garlic - 4 cloves

- Tomato paste - 1/4 cup

- Apple cider vinegar - 3 tbsp

- Paprika - 1 tsp

- Oregano (dried) - 1 tsp

- Thyme (dried) - 1 tsp

- A small handful of basil

Desired salt and pepper to taste

Instructions

1. With a cooking spray, line a large rimmed baking sheet and put it in an over 400 degrees preheated oven.

2.   Slice each tomato into four slices, remove the seeds inside the pepper and slice into eighths. Place the peppers, garlic cloves and tomatoes onto the prepared baking sheet and mist with an olive oil mister. Evenly sprinkle the paprika, oregano, thyme, and salt and pepper on top, then place in oven and roast for 30-35 minutes.

3.   In a large pot, heat the olive oil and add diced onions and sauté and leave until they begin to soften in about 2 minutes.

4.   Lower the heat and add roasted vegetables and garlic cloves, able cider vinegar, tomato paste, fresh basil, and two cups of water. Blend using the immersion blender until it gets smooth.

5.   Lower the heat further and add in the roasted vegetables and garlic cloves, tomato paste, able cider vinegar, fresh basil, and two cups of water, add water to achieve desired consistency.

6.   Add pepper and salt to taste and cover on low heat. Stir for about 20-30 minutes regularly.

7.   This homemade meal is sure to become your gateway. Savor the flavor of the roasted veggies and garlic.

Mushroom & Broccoli Soup

Total Time

Prep: 20 min. Cook: 45 min.

Makes

8 servings

Ingredients:

- 1 bundle broccoli (around 1-1/2 pounds)

- 1 tablespoon canola oil

- 1/2 pound cut crisp mushrooms

- 1 tablespoon diminished sodium soy sauce

- 2 medium carrots, finely slashed

- 2 celery ribs, finely slashed

- 1/4 cup finely slashed onion

- 1 garlic clove, minced

- 1 container (32 ounces) vegetable juices

- 2 cups of water

- 2 tablespoons lemon juice

Directions:

1. Cut broccoli florets into reduced down pieces. Strip and hack stalks.

2. In an enormous pot, heat oil over medium-high warmth; saute mushrooms until delicate, 4-6 minutes. Mix in soy sauce; expel from skillet.

3. In the same container, join broccoli stalks, carrots, celery, onion, garlic, soup, and water; heat to the point of boiling. Diminish heat; stew, revealed, until vegetables are relaxed, 25-30 minutes.

4. Puree soup utilizing a drenching blender. Or then again, cool marginally and puree the soup in a blender; come back to the dish. Mix in florets and mushrooms; heat to the point of boiling. Lessen warmth to medium; cook until broccoli is delicate, 8-10 minutes, blending infrequently. Mix in lemon juice.

Creamy Cauliflower Pakora Soup

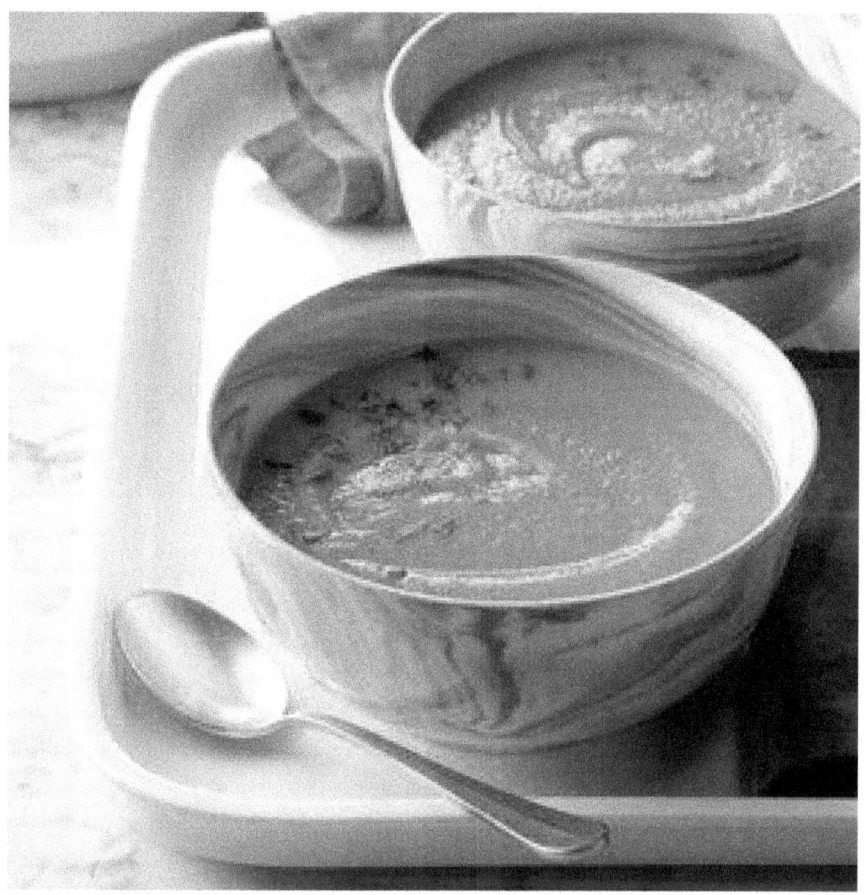

Total Time

Prep: 20 min. Cook: 20 min.

Makes

8 servings (3 quarts)

Ingredients:

- 1 huge head cauliflower, cut into little florets

- 5 medium potatoes, stripped and diced

- 1 huge onion, diced

- 4 medium carrots, stripped and diced

- 2 celery ribs, diced

- 1 container (32 ounces) vegetable stock

- 1 teaspoon garam masala

- 1 teaspoon garlic powder

- 1 teaspoon ground coriander

- 1 teaspoon ground turmeric

- 1 teaspoon ground cumin

- 1 teaspoon pepper

- 1 teaspoon salt

- 1/2 teaspoon squashed red pepper chips Water or extra vegetable stock New cilantro leaves

- Lime wedges, discretionary

Directions

1. In a Dutch stove over medium-high warmth, heat initial 14 fixings to the point of boiling. Cook and mix until vegetables are delicate, around 20 minutes. Expel from heat; cool marginally. Procedure in groups in a blender or nourishment processor until smooth. Modify consistency as wanted with water (or extra stock). Sprinkle with new cilantro. Serve hot, with lime wedges whenever wanted.

2. Stop alternative: Before including cilantro, solidify cooled soup in cooler compartments. To utilize, in part defrost in cooler medium-term. Warmth through in a pan, blending every so often and including a little water if fundamental. Sprinkle with cilantro. Whenever wanted, present with lime wedges.

Garden Vegetable and Herb Soup

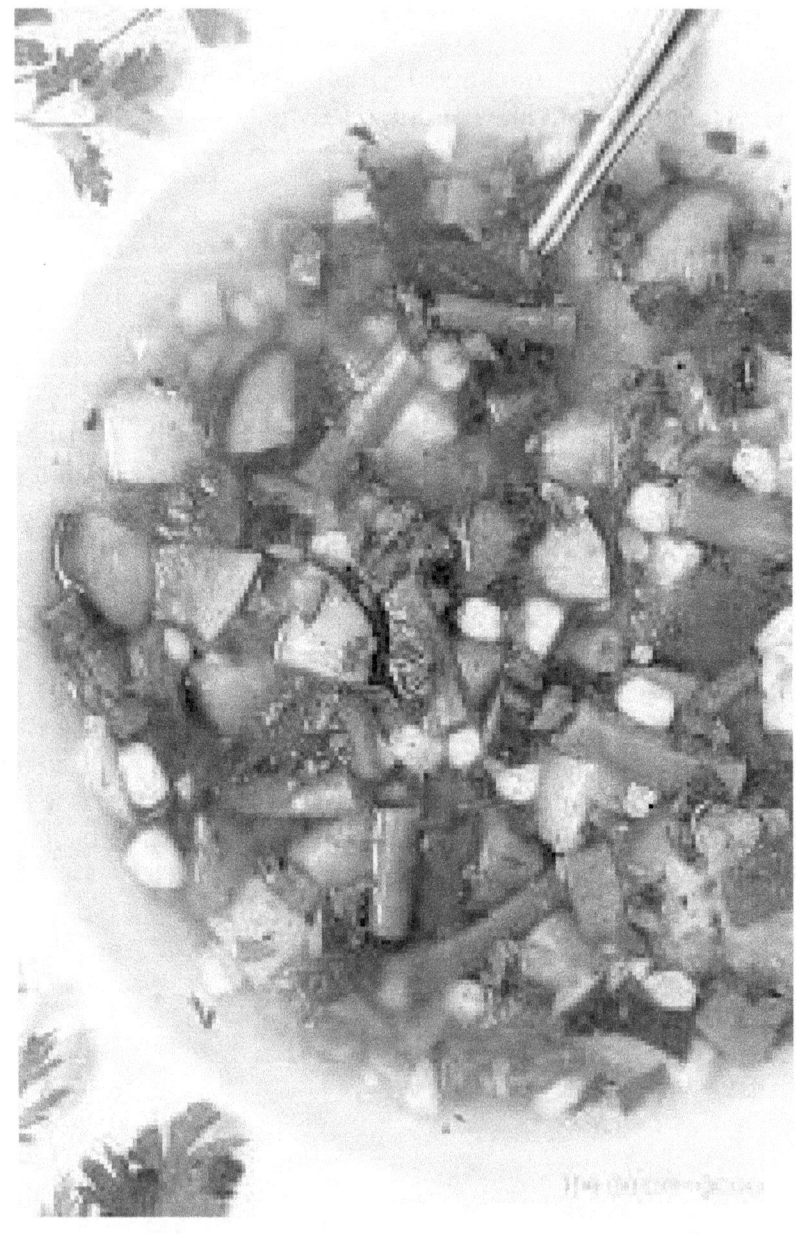

Total Time

Prep: 20 min. Cook: 30 min.

Makes

8 servings (2 quarts)

Ingredients:

- 2 tablespoons olive oil

- 2 medium onions, hacked

- 2 huge carrots, cut

- 1 pound red potatoes (around 3 medium), cubed

- 2 cups of water

- 1 can (14-1/2 ounces) diced tomatoes in sauce

- 1-1/2 cups vegetable soup

- 1-1/2 teaspoons garlic powder

- 1 teaspoon dried basil

- 1/2 teaspoon salt

- 1/2 teaspoon paprika

- 1/4 teaspoon dill weed

- 1/4 teaspoon pepper

- 1 medium yellow summer squash, split and cut

- 1 medium zucchini, split and cut

Directions:

1. In a huge pan, heat oil over medium warmth. Include onions and carrots; cook and mix until onions are delicate, 4-6 minutes. Include potatoes and cook 2 minutes. Mix in water, tomatoes, juices, and seasonings. Heat to the point of boiling. Diminish heat; stew, revealed, until potatoes and carrots are delicate, 9 minutes.

2. Include yellow squash and zucchini; cook until vegetables are delicate, 9 minutes longer. Serve or, whenever wanted, puree blend in clusters, including extra stock until wanted consistency is accomplished.

Super-easy Chicken Noodle Soup

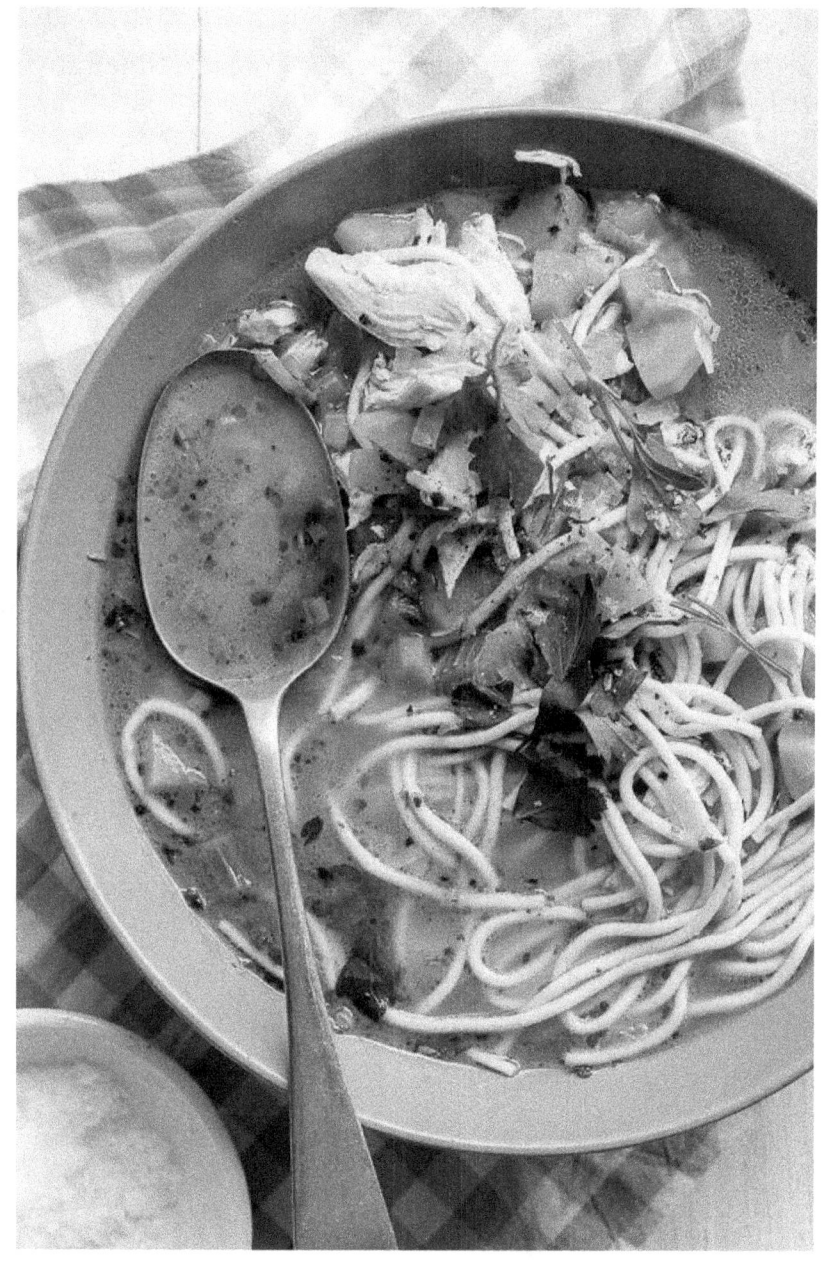

SmartPoints value: Green plan - 3SP, Blue plan - 2SP, Purple plan - 2SP

Total Time: 32 min, Prep time: 12 min, Cooking time: 20 min, Serves: 8

Nutritional value: Calories - 351.3, Carbs - 37.3g, Fat - 4.5g, Protein - 39.7g

In this recipe, I will make it easy for you to prepare a hearty soup for the whole family, all with just one pot. A big cup of 1 1/2 portion has only two SmartPoints value, so it's perfect for lunch, either to take to work or for your child's lunchbox, too.

Unlike other recipes like it, this one will be ready in just 32 minutes, not hours!

Now, pick up some ZeroPoint chicken breasts, frozen vegetables, a box of pasta, chicken broth, and a few more bits and pieces, and let's get you started on this family delight.

Ingredients

Black pepper - ¼ tsp

- Chicken breast(s) (cooked) - 6 oz, chopped (skinless, boneless)

- Salted butter - 2 tsp

- Onion(s) (uncooked) - 1 large, well chopped

- Table salt - 1½ tsp, divided

- Chicken broth (reduced-sodium) - 64 oz

- Pasta (uncooked) - 4 oz, small shape such as ditalini (about 1 cup)

- Mixed vegetables (frozen) - 10 oz, such as peas, green beans, and carrots

- Tomatoes (canned) - 15 oz, petite cut, rinsed and drained

- Parmesan cheese (grated) - 1 Tbsp

- Lemon juice (fresh) - 2 tsp

- Fresh chives - ¼ cup(s), chopped (optional)

Instructions

1. Melt two teaspoons of butter in a large stockpot over medium-low heat.

2.	Add well-chopped onion and 1/2 teaspoon of salt, then cook, often stirring, until the onion is soft and translucent; about 10 minutes.
3.	Add the broth in the chicken and increase the heat to high, then bring it to a boil.

4.	Put in the pasta, frozen vegetables, and tomatoes, then cook until pasta is soft; about 7 minutes.

5.	Stir in the chicken, lemon juice, cheese, remaining one teaspoon of salt, black pepper, and chives, then cook one more minute to heat through.

Hearty Ginger Soup

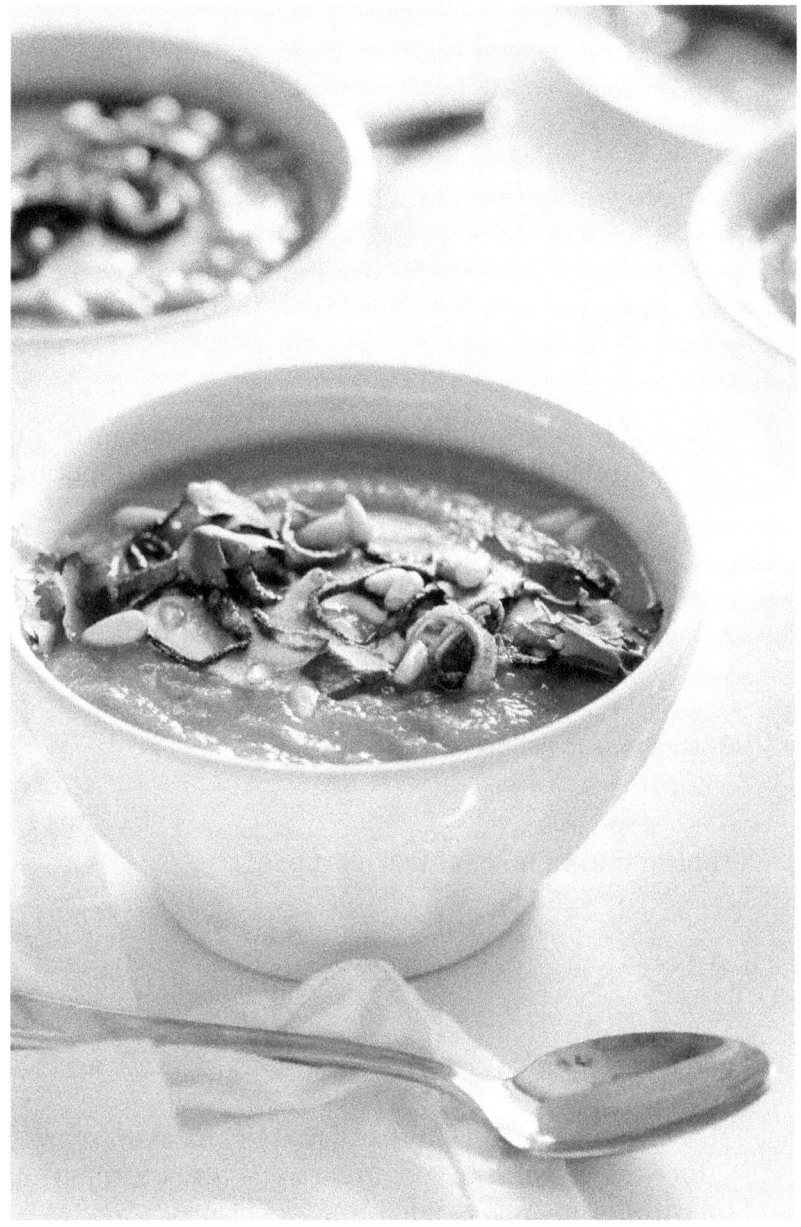

Serving: 4

Prep Time: 5 minutes

Cook Time: 5 minutes

Ingredients:

- 3 cups coconut almond milk

- 2 cups water

- ½ pound boneless chicken breast halves, cut into chunks 3 tablespoons fresh ginger root, minced 2 tablespoons fish sauce

- ¼ cup fresh lime juice

- 2 tablespoons green onions, sliced

- 1 tablespoon fresh cilantro, chopped

How To:

1. Take a saucepan and add coconut almond milk and water.
2. Bring the mixture to a boil and add the chicken strips.
3. Reduce the warmth to medium and simmer for 3 minutes.
4. Stir within the ginger, juice , and fish sauce.
5. Sprinkle a couple of green onions and cilantro.

6. Serve!

Nutrition (Per Serving)

Calories: 415

Fat: 39g

Carbohydrates: 8g

Protein: 14g

Tasty Tofu and Mushroom Soup

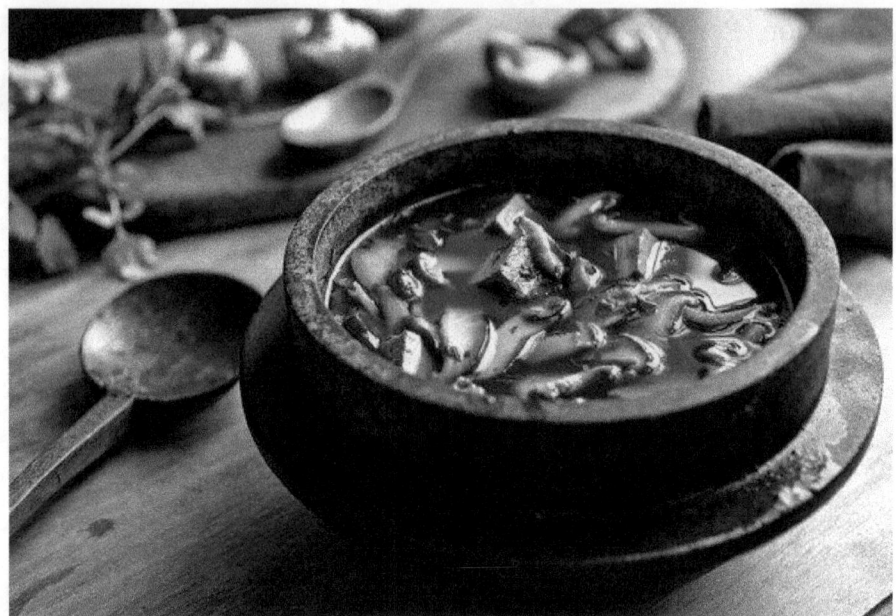

Serving: 8

Prep Time: 10 minutes

Cook Time: 10 minutes

Ingredients:

- 3 cups prepared dashi stock

- ¼ cup shiitake mushrooms, sliced

- 1 tablespoon miso paste

- 1 tablespoon coconut aminos

- 1/8 cup cubed soft tofu

1 green onion, diced

How To:

1. Take a saucepan and add stock, bring back a boil.
2. Add mushrooms, cook for 4 minutes.
3. Take a bowl and add coconut aminos, miso paste and blend well.
4. Pour the mixture into stock and let it cook for six minutes on simmer.
5. Add diced green onions and enjoy!

Nutrition (Per Serving)

Calories: 100

Fat: 4g

Carbohydrates: 5g

Protein: 11

Ingenious Eggplant Soup

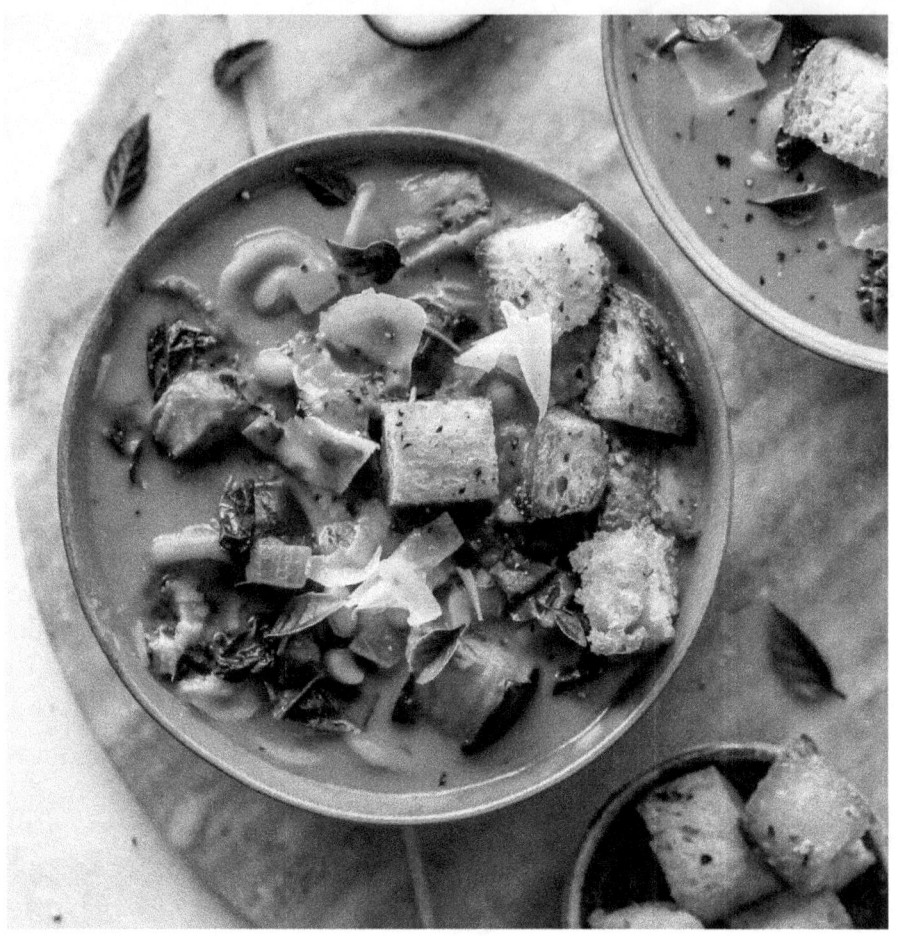

Serving: 8

Prep Time: 20 minutes

Cook Time: 15 minutes

Ingredients:

- 1 large eggplant, washed and cubed

- 1 tomato, seeded and chopped
- 1 small onion, diced
- 2 tablespoons parsley, chopped
- 2 tablespoons extra virgin olive oil
- 2 tablespoons distilled white vinegar
- ½ cup parmesan cheese, crumbled Sunflower seeds as needed

How To:

1. Pre-heat your outdoor grill to medium-high.
2. Pierce the eggplant a couple of times employing a knife/fork.
3. Cook the eggplants on your grill for about quarter-hour until they're charred.
4. forgot and permit them to chill .
5. Remove the skin from the eggplant and dice the pulp.
6. Transfer the pulp to a bowl and add parsley, onion, tomato, olive oil, feta cheese and vinegar.
7. Mix well and chill for 1 hour.
8. Season with sunflower seeds and enjoy!

Nutrition (Per Serving)

Calories: 99

Fat: 7g

Carbohydrates: 7g

Protein: 3.4g

Loving Cauliflower Soup

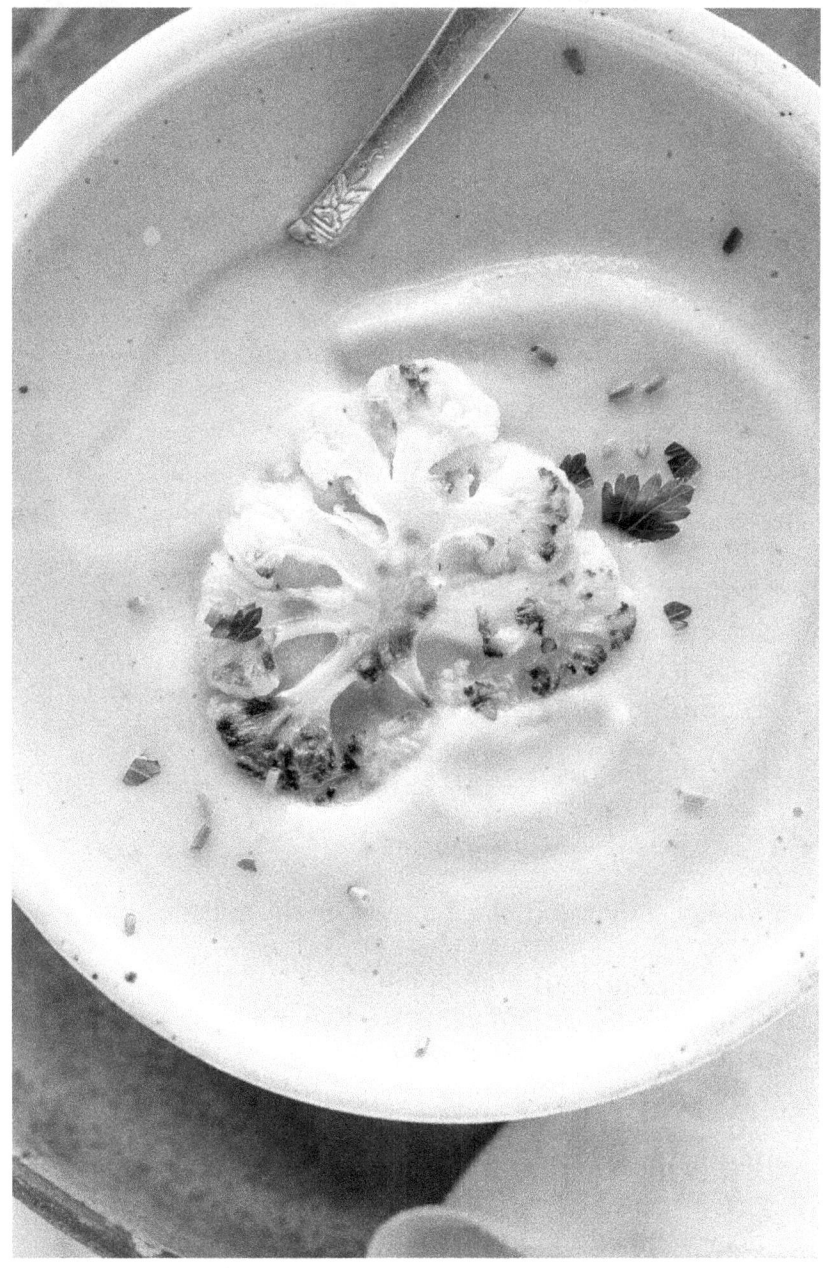

Serving: 6

Prep Time: 10 minutes

Cook Time: 10 minutes

Ingredients:

- 4 cups vegetable stock
- 1-pound cauliflower, trimmed and chopped
- 7 ounces Kite ricotta/cashew cheese
- 4 ounces almond butter
- Sunflower seeds and pepper to taste

How To:

1. Take a skillet and place it over medium heat.
2. Add almond butter and melt.
3. Add cauliflower and sauté for two minutes.
4. Add stock and convey mix to a boil.
5. Cook until cauliflower is hard .
6. Stir in cheese , sunflower seeds and pepper.
7. Puree the combination using an immersion blender.
8. Serve and enjoy!

Nutrition (Per Serving)

Calories: 143

Fat: 16g

Carbohydrates: 6g

Protein: 3.4g

Simple Garlic and Lemon Soup

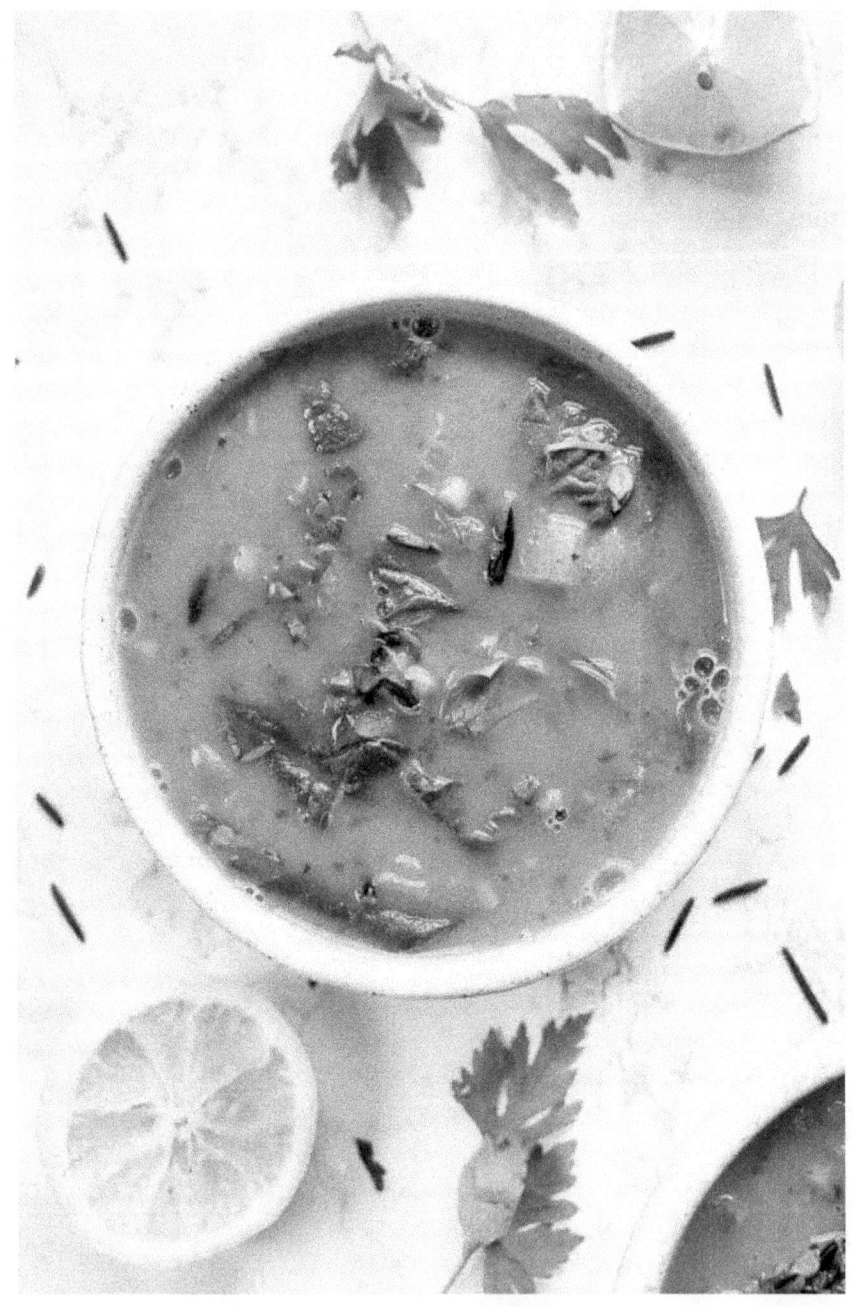

Serving: 3

Prep Time: 10 minutes

Cook Time: nil

Ingredients:

- 1 avocado, pitted and chopped
- 1 cucumber, chopped
- 2 bunches spinach
- 1 ½ cups watermelon, chopped
- 1 bunch cilantro, roughly chopped
- Juice from 2 lemons
- ½ cup coconut amines
- ½ cup lime juice

How To:

1. Add cucumber, avocado to your blender and pulse well.

2. Add cilantro, spinach and watermelon and blend.
3. Add lemon, juice and coconut amino.
4. Pulse a couple of more times.
5. Transfer to bowl and enjoy!

Nutrition (Per Serving)

Calories: 100

Fat: 7g

Carbohydrates: 6g

Protein: 3g

Healthy Cucumber Soup

Serving: 4

Prep Time: 14 minutes

Cook Time: Nil

Ingredients:

- 2 tablespoons garlic, minced

- 4 cups English cucumbers, peeled and diced ½ cup onions, diced

- 1 tablespoon lemon juice 1 ½ cups vegetable broth ½ teaspoon sunflower seeds ¼ teaspoon red pepper flakes

- ¼ cup parsley, diced

- ½ cup Greek yogurt, plain

How To:

1. Add the listed ingredients to a blender and blend to emulsify (keep aside ½ cup of chopped cucumbers).

2. Blend until smooth.
3. Divide the soup amongst 4 servings and top with extra cucumbers.

4. Enjoy chilled!

Nutrition (Per Serving)

Calories: 371

Fat: 36g

Carbohydrates: 8g

Protein: 4g

Mushroom Cream Soup

Serving: 4

Prep Time: 5 minutes

Cook Time: 30 minutes

Ingredients:

- 1 tablespoon olive oil

- ½ large onion, diced

- 20 ounces mushrooms, sliced

- 6 garlic cloves, minced

- 2 cups vegetable broth

- 1 cup coconut cream

- ¾ teaspoon sunflower seeds

- ¼ teaspoon black pepper

- 1 cup almond milk

How To:

1. Take an outsized sized pot and place it over medium heat.

2. Add onion and mushrooms to the vegetable oil and sauté for 10-15 minutes.
3. confirm to stay stirring it from time to time until browned evenly.

4. Add garlic and sauté for 10 minutes more.
5. Add vegetable broth, coconut milk , almond milk[MOU6], black

pepper and sunflower seeds.

6. Bring it to a boil and lower the temperature to low.
7. Simmer for quarter-hour .
8. Use an immersion blender to puree the mixture.
9. Enjoy!

Nutrition (Per Serving)

Calories: 200

Fat: 17g

Carbohydrates: 5g

Protein: 4g

Curious Roasted Garlic Soup

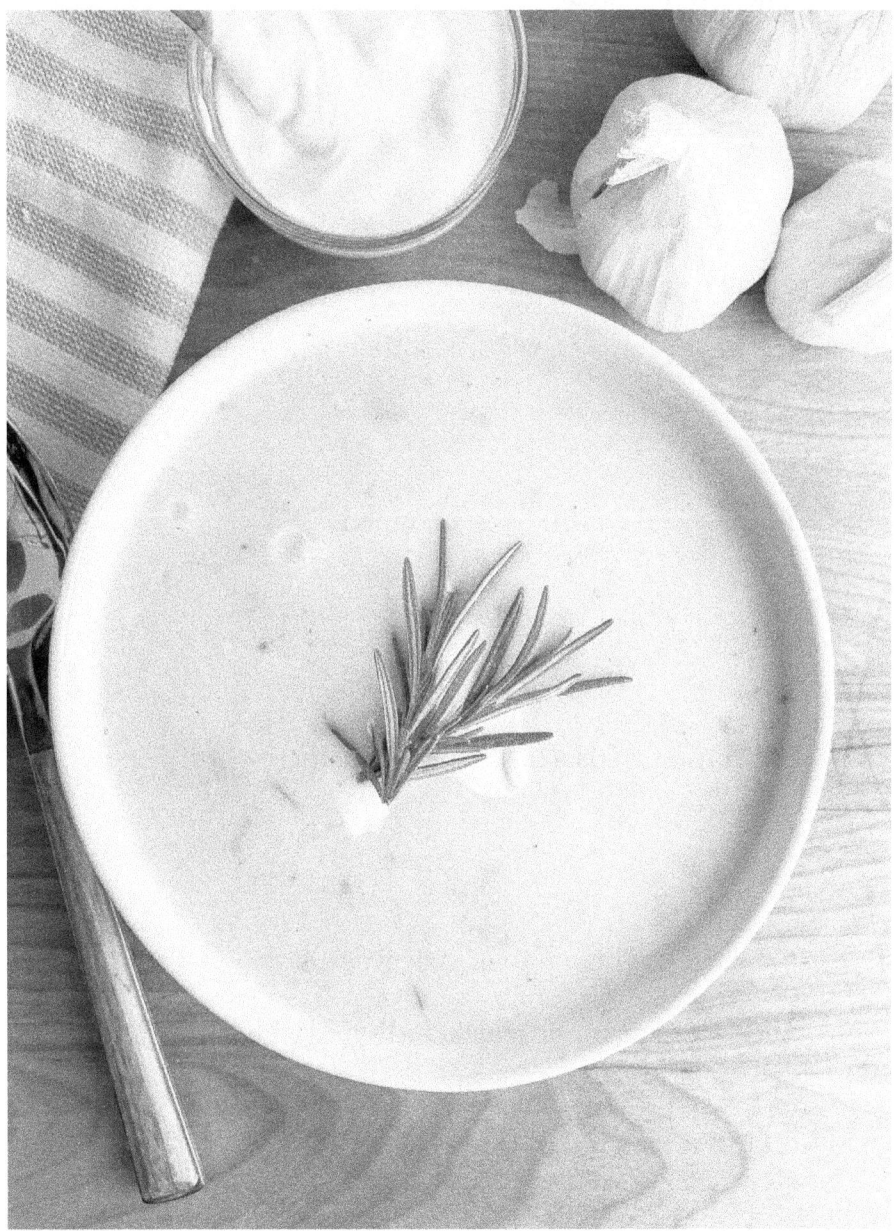

Serving: 10

Prep Time: 10 minutes

Cook Time: 60 minutes

Ingredients:

- 1 tablespoon olive oil
- 2 bulbs garlic, peeled
- 3 shallots, chopped
- 1 large head cauliflower, chopped
- 6 cups vegetable broth
- Sunflower seeds and pepper to taste

How To:

1. Pre-heat your oven to 400 degrees F.
2. Slice ¼ inch top of garlic bulb and place it in aluminum foil.
3. Grease with vegetable oil and roast in oven for 35 minutes.
4. Squeeze flesh out of the roasted garlic.
5. Heat oil in saucepan and add shallots, sauté for six minutes.
6. Add garlic and remaining ingredients.
7. Cover pan and reduce heat to low.
8. Let it cook for 15-20 minutes.

9. Use an immersion blender to puree the mixture. 10. Season soup

with sunflower seeds and pepper.

10. Serve and enjoy!

Nutrition (Per Serving)

Calories: 142

Fat: 8g

Carbohydrates: 3.4g

Protein: 4g

Amazing Roasted Carrot Soup

Serving: 4

Prep Time: 10 minutes

Cook Time: 50 minutes

Ingredients:

- 8 large carrots, washed and peeled

- 6 tablespoons olive oil

- 1-quart broth

- Cayenne pepper to taste

- Sunflower seeds and pepper to taste

How To:

1. Pre-heat your oven to 425 degrees F.

2. Take a baking sheet and add carrots, drizzle vegetable oil and roast for 30-45 minutes.
3. Put roasted carrots into blender and add broth, puree.
4. Pour into saucepan and warmth soup.
5. Season with sunflower seeds, pepper and cayenne.
6. Drizzle vegetable oil .

7. Serve and enjoy!

Nutrition (Per Serving)

Calories: 222

Fat: 18g

Net Carbohydrates: 7g

Protein: 5g

Simple Pumpkin Soup

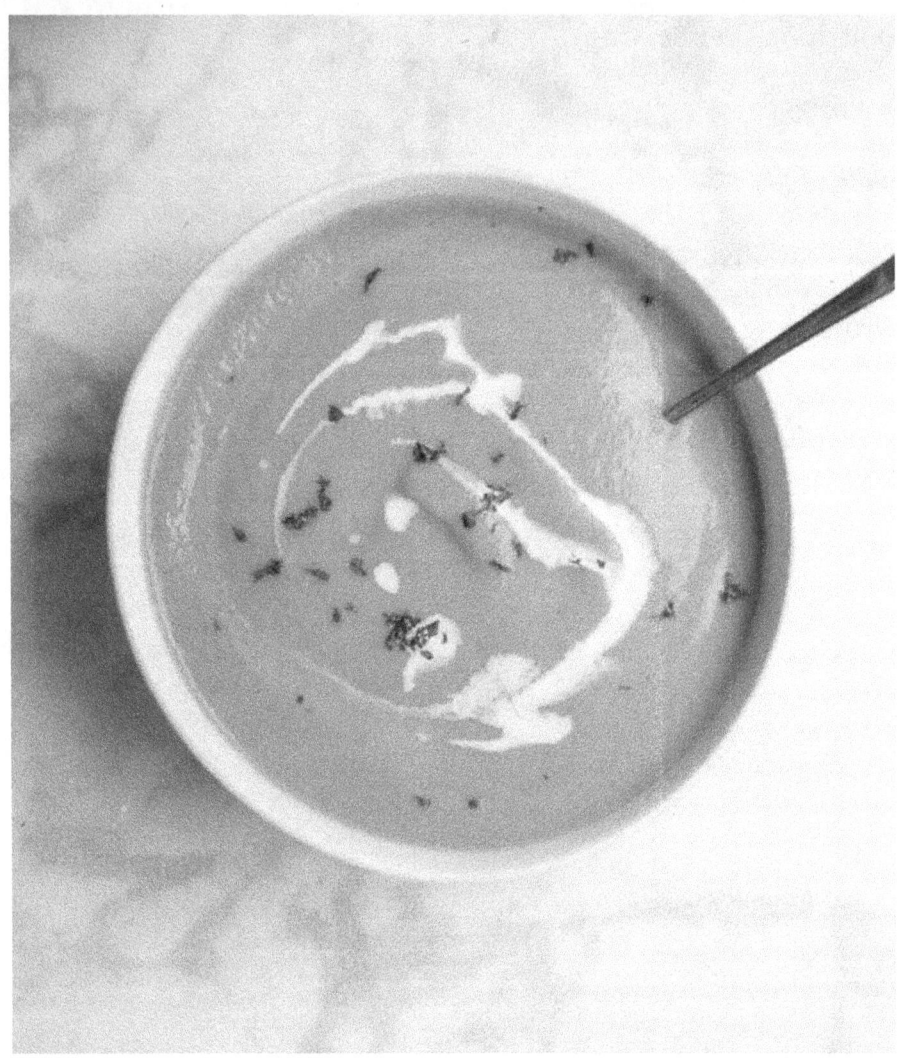

Serving: 4

Prep Time: 5 minutes

Cook Time: 6-8 hours

Ingredients:

- 1 small pumpkin, halved, peeled, seeds removed, cubed
- 2 cups chicken broth
- 1 cup coconut milk
- Pepper and thyme to taste

How To:

1. Add all the ingredients to a crockpot.
2. Close the lid.
3. Cook for 6-8 hours on low.
4. Make a smooth puree by employing a blender.
5. Garnish with roasted seeds.
6. Serve and enjoy!

Nutrition (Per Serving)

Calories: 60

Fat: 2g

Net Carbohydrates: 10g

Protein: 3g

Coconut Avocado Soup

Serving: 4

Prep Time: 5 minutes

Cook Time: 5-10 minutes

Ingredients:

- 2 cups vegetable stock

- 2 teaspoons Thai green curry paste

- Pepper as needed

- 1 avocado, chopped

- 1 tablespoon cilantro, chopped

- Lime wedges

- 1 cup coconut milk

How To:

1. Add milk, avocado, curry paste, pepper to blender and blend.

2. Take a pan and place it over medium heat.
3. Add mixture and warmth , simmer for five minutes.
4. Stir in seasoning, cilantro and simmer for 1 minute.
5. Serve and enjoy!

Nutrition (Per Serving)

Calories: 250

Fat: 30g

Net Carbohydrates: 2g

Protein: 4g

Coconut Arugula Soup

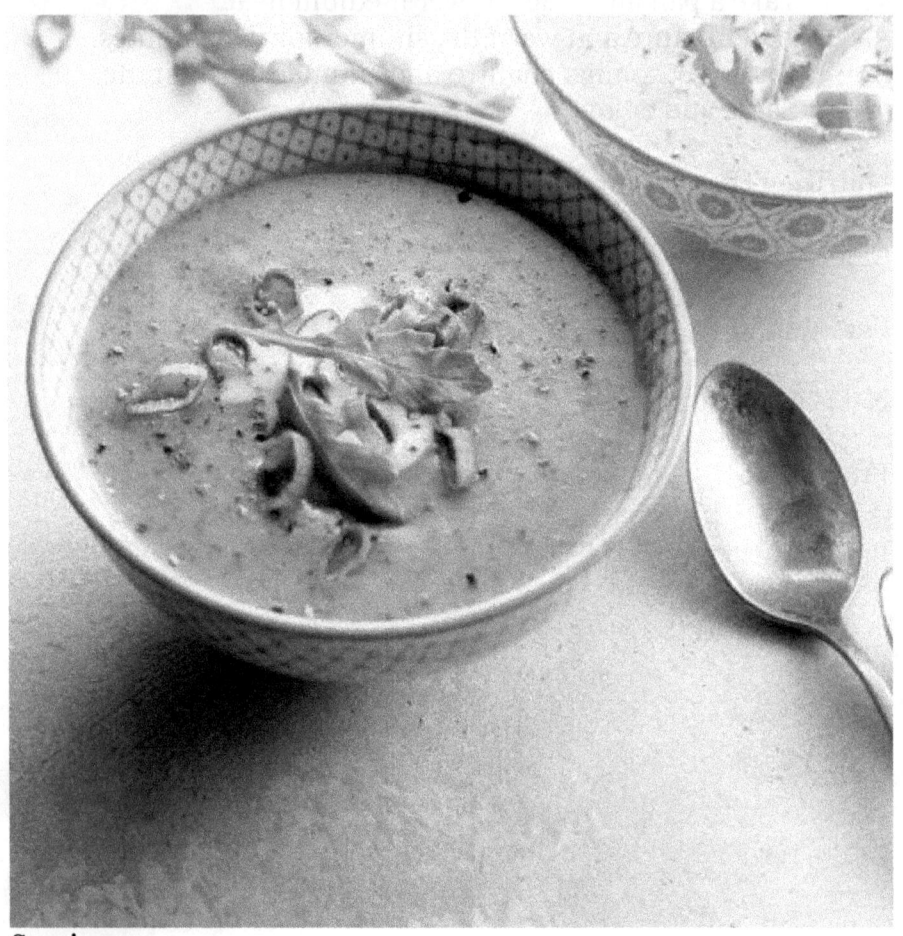

Serving: 4

Prep Time: 5 minutes

Cook Time: 5-10 minutes

Ingredients:

Black pepper as needed

- 1 tablespoon olive oil

- 2 tablespoons chives, chopped

- 2 garlic cloves, minced

- 10 ounces baby arugula

- 2 tablespoons tarragon, chopped

- 4 tablespoons coconut milk yogurt

- 6 cups chicken stock

- 2 tablespoons mint, chopped

- 1 onion, chopped
- ½ cup coconut milk

How To:

1. Take a saucepan and place it over medium-high heat, add oil and let it heat up.

2. Add onion and garlic and fry for five minutes.
3. Stir available and reduce the warmth, let it simmer.
4. Stir in tarragon, arugula, mint, parsley and cook for six minutes.

5. Mix in seasoning , chives, coconut yogurt and serve.
6. Enjoy!

Nutrition (Per Serving)

Calories: 180

Fat: 14g

Net Carbohydrates: 20g

Protein: 2g

Awesome Cabbage Soup

Serving: 3

Prep Time: 7 minutes

Cook Time: 25 minutes

Ingredients:

- 3 cups non-fat beef stock
- 2 garlic cloves, minced
- 1 tablespoon tomato paste
- 2 cups cabbage, chopped
- ½ yellow onion
- ½ cup carrot, chopped
- ½ cup green beans
- ½ cup zucchini, chopped
- ½ teaspoon basil

- ½ teaspoon oregano

- Sunflower seeds and pepper as needed

How To:

1. Grease a pot with non-stick cooking spray.
2. Place it over medium heat and permit the oil to heat up.
3. Add onions, carrots, and garlic and sauté for five minutes.
4. Add broth, ingredient , green beans, cabbage, basil, oregano, sunflower seeds, and pepper.
5. Bring the entire mix to a boil and reduce the warmth , simmer for 5-10 minutes until all veggies are tender.
6. Add zucchini and simmer for five minutes more.
7. Sever hot and enjoy!

Nutrition (Per Serving)

Calories: 22

Fat: 0g

Carbohydrates: 5g

Protein: 1g

Ginger Zucchini Avocado Soup

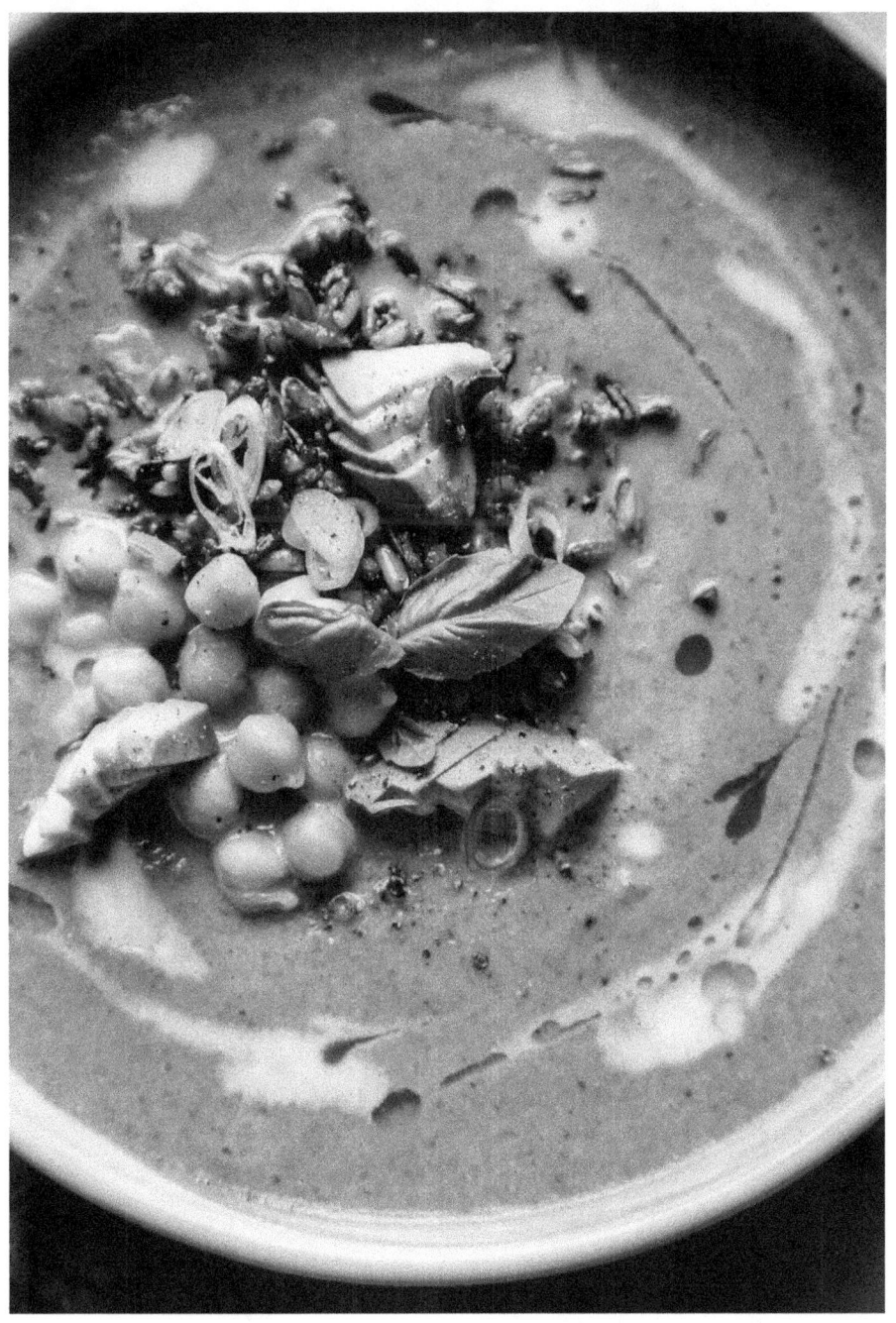

Serving: 3

Prep Time: 7 minutes

Cook Time: 25 minutes

Ingredients:

- 1 red bell pepper, chopped

- 1 big avocado

- 1 teaspoon ginger, grated

- Pepper as needed

- 2 tablespoons avocado oil

- 4 scallions, chopped

- 1 tablespoon lemon juice

- 29 ounces vegetable stock

- 1 garlic clove, minced

- 2 zucchini, chopped

- 1 cup water

How To:

1. Take a pan and place over medium heat, add onion and fry for 3 minutes.

2. Stir in ginger, garlic and cook for 1 minute.
3. Mix in seasoning, zucchini stock, water and boil for 10 minutes.

4. Remove soup from fire and let it sit, blend in avocado and blend using an immersion blender.
5. Heat over low heat for a short time .
6. Adjust your seasoning and add juice , bell pepper.
7. Serve and enjoy!

Nutrition (Per Serving)

Calories: 155

Fat: 11g

Carbohydrates: 10g

Protein: 7g

Greek Lemon and Chicken Soup

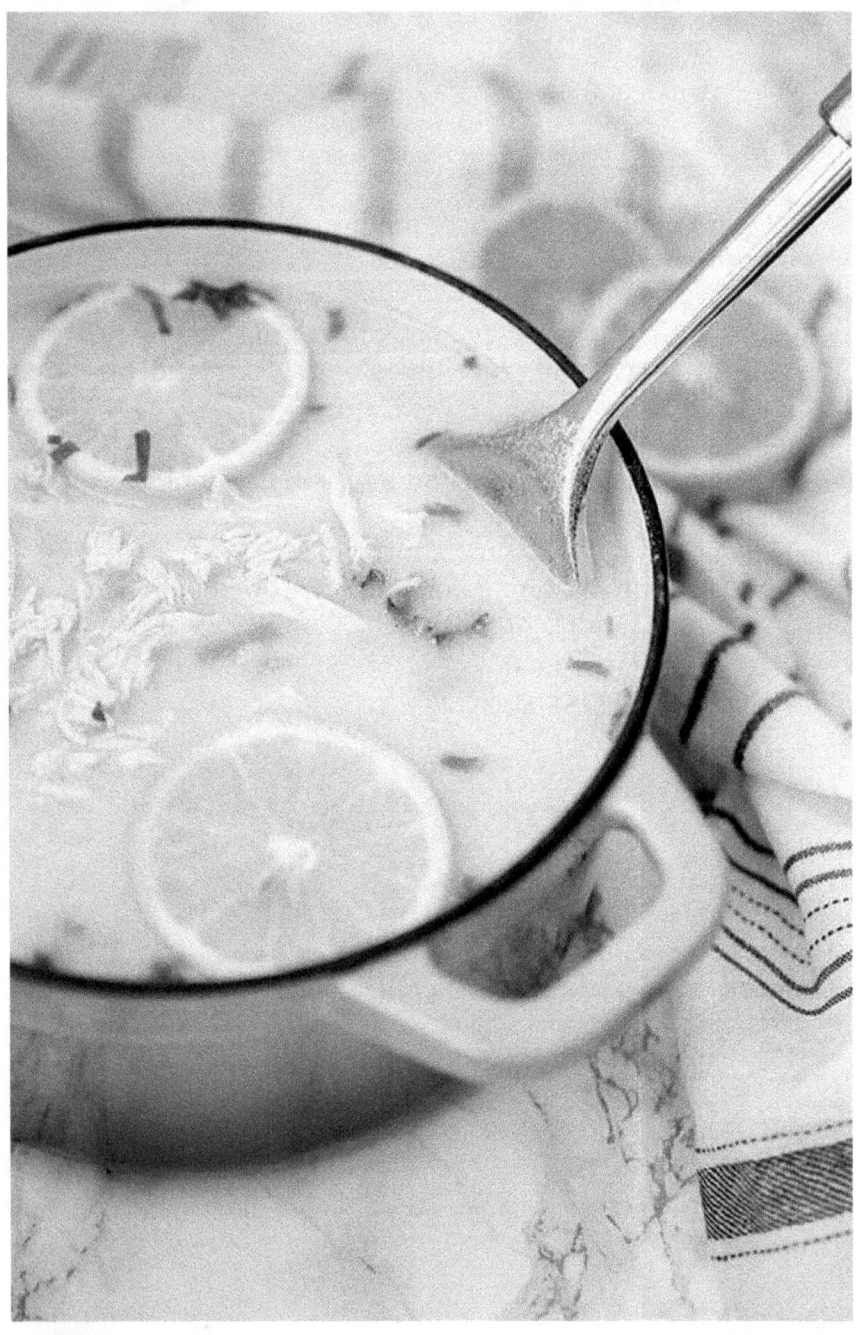

Serving: 4

Prep Time: 15 minutes

Cook Time: 30 minutes

Ingredients:

- 2 cups cooked chicken, chopped

- 2 medium carrots, chopped

- ½ cup onion, chopped ¼ cup lemon juice 1 clove garlic, minced

- 1 can cream of chicken soup, fat-free and low sodium

- 2 cans chicken broth, fat-free

- ¼ teaspoon ground black pepper

- 2/3 cup long-grain rice

- 2 tablespoons parsley, snipped

How To:

1. Add all of the listed ingredients to a pot (except rice and parsley).
2. Season with sunflower seeds and pepper.
3. Bring the combination to a overboil medium-high heat.
4. Stir in rice and set heat to medium.
5. Simmer for 20 minutes until rice is tender.
6. Garnish parsley and enjoy!

Nutrition (Per Serving)

Calories: 582

Fat: 33g

Carbohydrates: 35g

Protein: 32g

Morning Peach

Serving: 4

Prep Time: 10 minutes

Cook Time: 5 minutes

Ingredients:

- 6 small peaches, cored and cut into wedges ¼ cup coconut sugar

- 2 tablespoons almond butter

- ¼ teaspoon almond extract

How To:

1. Take alittle pan and add peaches, sugar, butter and flavor.
2. Toss well.
3. Cook over medium-high heat for five minutes, divide the combination into bowls and serve.
4. Enjoy!

Nutrition (Per Serving)

Calories: 198

Fat: 2g

Carbohydrates: 11g

Protein: 8g

Garlic and Pumpkin Soup

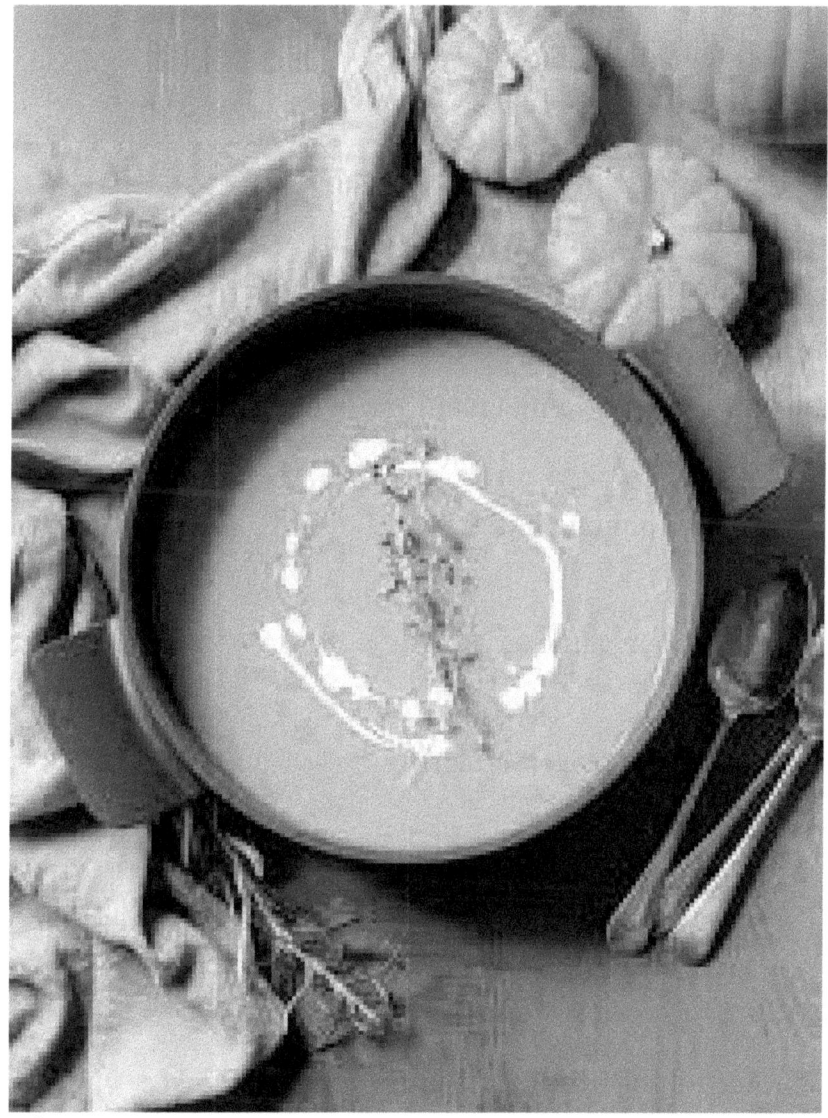

Serving: 4

Prep Time: 10 minutes

Cook Time: 5 hours

Ingredients:

- 1-pound pumpkin chunks
- 1 onion, diced
- 2 cups vegetable stock
- 1 2/3 cups coconut cream
- ½ stick almond butter
- 1 teaspoon garlic, crushed
- 1 teaspoon ginger, crushed
- Pepper to taste

How To:

1. Add all the ingredients into your Slow Cooker.
2. Cook for 4-6 hours on high.
3. Puree the soup by using an immersion blender.
4. Serve and enjoy!

Nutrition (Per Serving)

Calories: 235

Fat: 21g

Carbohydrates: 11g

Protein: 2g

Butternut and Garlic Soup

Serving: 4

Prep Time: 5 minutes

Cook Time: 35 minutes

Ingredients:

- 4 cups butternut squash, cubed
- 4 cups vegetable broth, stock
- ½ cup low fat cream
- 2 garlic cloves, chopped
- Pepper to taste

How To:

1. Add butternut squash, garlic cloves, broth, salt and pepper during a large pot.
2. Place the pot over medium heat and canopy with the lid.
3. Bring back boil then reduce the temperature.
4. Let it simmer for 30-35 minutes.[MOU7]
5. Blend the soup for 1-2 minutes until you get a smooth mixture.

6. Stir the cream through the soup.
7. Serve and enjoy!

Nutrition (Per Serving)

Calories: 180
Fat: 14g

Carbohydrates: 21g

Protein: 3g

Minty Avocado Soup

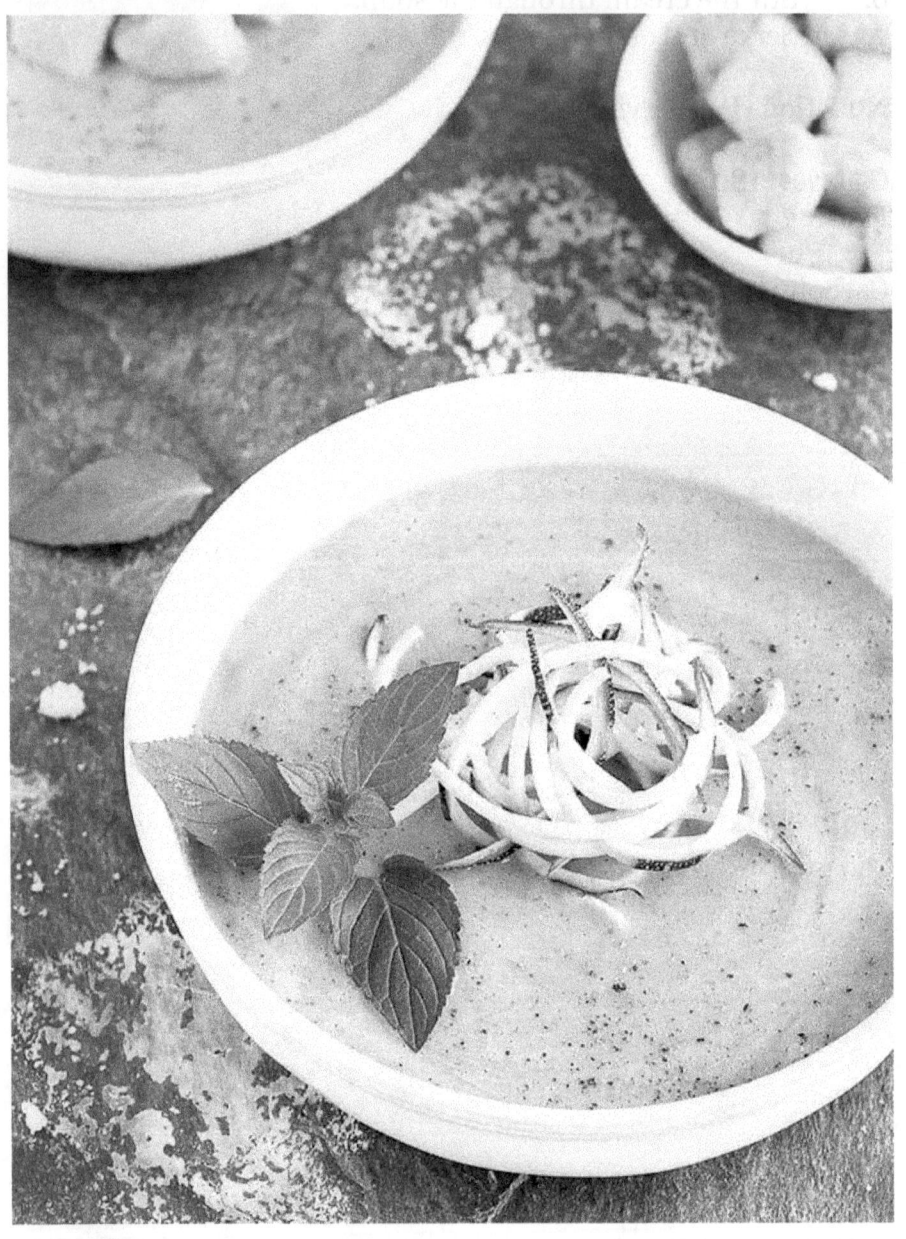

Serving: 4

Prep Time: 10 minutes + Chill time

Cook Time: nil

Ingredients:

- 1 avocado, ripe
- 1 cup coconut almond milk, chilled
- 2 romaine lettuce leaves
- 20 mint leaves, fresh
- 1 tablespoon lime juice
- Sunflower seeds, to taste

How To:

1. Activate your slow cooker and add all the ingredients into it.
2. Mix them during a kitchen appliance .
3. Make a smooth mixture.
4. Let it chill for 10 minutes.
5. Serve and enjoy!

Nutrition (Per Serving)

Calories: 280

Fat: 26g

Carbohydrates: 12g

Protein: 4g

Celery, Cucumber and Zucchini Soup

Serving: 2

Prep Time: 10 minutes + Chill time

Cook Time: nil

Ingredients:

- 3 celery stalks, chopped

- 7 ounces cucumber, cubed

- 1 tablespoon olive oil

- 2/5 cup fresh cream, 30%, low fat

- 1 red bell pepper, chopped

- 1 tablespoon dill, chopped

- 10 ½ ounces zucchini, cubed

- Sunflower seeds and pepper, to taste

How To:

1. Put the vegetables during a juicer and juice.

2. Then mix within the vegetable oil and fresh cream.
3. Season with sauce and pepper.
4. Garnish with dill.

5. Serve it chilled and enjoy!

Nutrition (Per Serving)
Calories: 325

Fat: 32g

Carbohydrates: 10g

Protein: 4g

Rosemary and Thyme Cucumber Soup

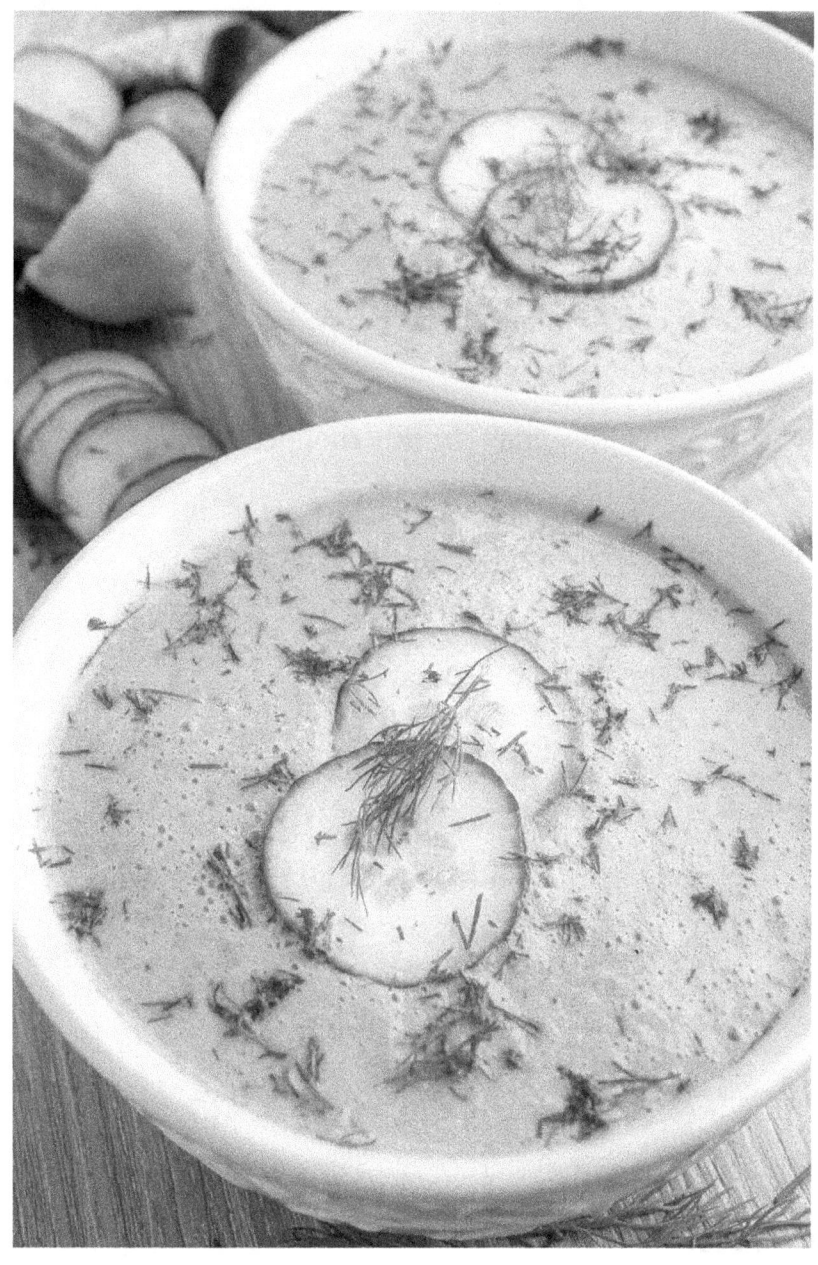

Serving: 3

Prep Time: 10 minutes + Chill time

Cook Time: nil

Ingredients:

- 4 cups vegetable broth
- 1 teaspoon thyme, freshly chopped
- 1 teaspoon rosemary, freshly chopped
- 2 cucumbers, sliced1 cup low fat cream
- 1 pinch of sunflower seeds

How To:

1. Take an outsized bowl and add all the ingredients.
2. Whisk well.
3. Blend until smooth by using an immersion blender.
4. Let it chill for 1 hour.
5. Serve and enjoy!

Nutrition (Per Serving)

Calories: 111

Fat: 8g

Carbohydrates: 4g

Protein: 5g

Guacamole Soup

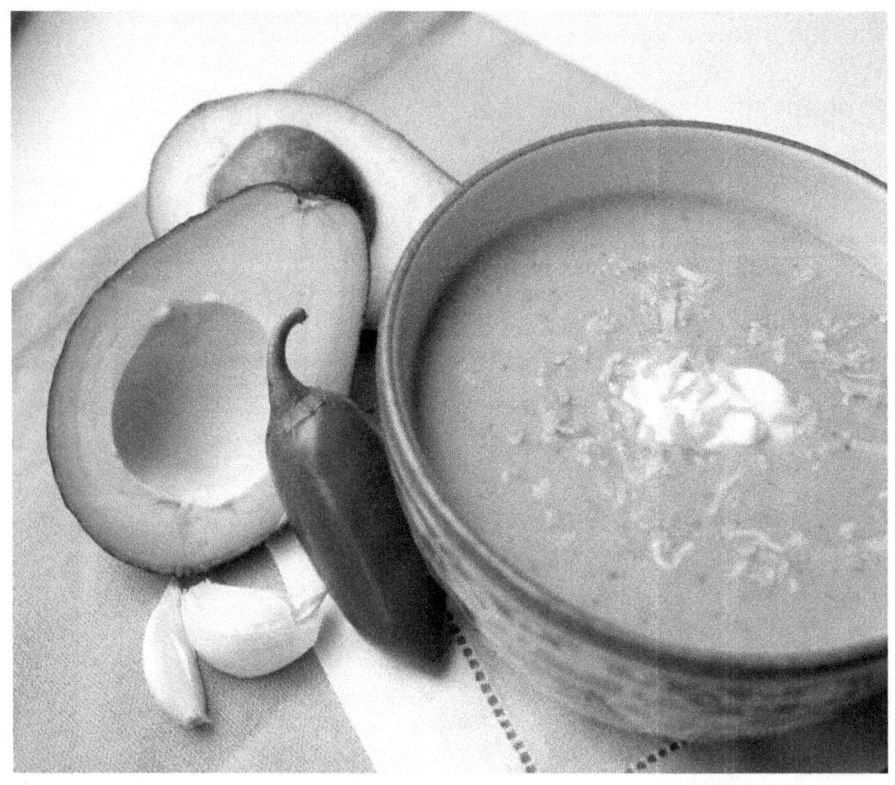

Serving: 3

Prep Time: 10 minute + Chill time

Cook Time: nil

Ingredients:

- 3 cups vegetable broth 2 ripe avocados, pitted ½ cup cilantro, freshly chopped

- 1 tomato, chopped

- ½ cup low fat cream

- Sunflower seeds & black pepper, to taste

How To:

1. Add all the ingredients into a blender.
2. Blend until creamy by using an immersion blender.
3. Let it chill for 1 hour.
4. Serve and enjoy!

Nutrition (Per Serving)

Calories: 289

Fat: 26g

Carbohydrates: 5g

Protein: 10g

Cucumber and Zucchini Soup

Serving: 3

Prep Time: 10 minutes + Chill time

Cook Time: nil

Ingredients:

- 2 tablespoons olive oil
- 1 tablespoon fresh dill
- 2/5 cup fresh cream
- 7 ounces cucumber, cubed
- 10 ½ zucchini, cubed
- 1 red pepper, chopped
- 3 celery stalks, chopped
- Sunflower seeds and pepper to taste

How To:

1. Add all the veggies during a juice and make a smooth juice.
2. Mix within the fresh cream and vegetable oil .
3. Season with pepper and sunflower seeds.
4. Garnish with dill.
5. Serve chilled and enjoy!

Nutrition (Per Serving)

Calories: 100

Fat: 8g

Carbohydrates: 4g

Protein: 2g

Crockpot Pumpkin Soup

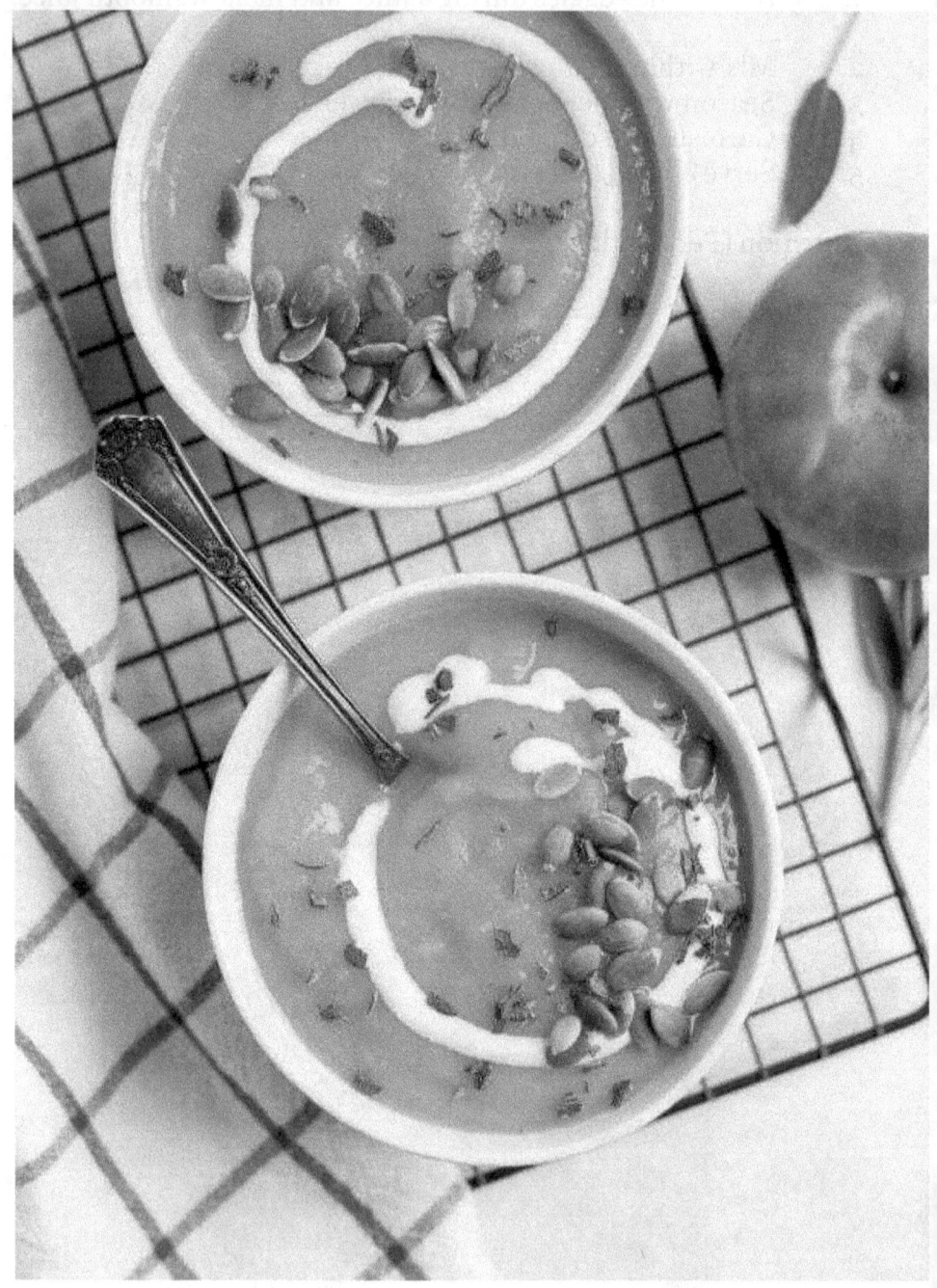

Serving: 3

Prep Time: 10 minute

Cook Time: 6-8 hours

Ingredients:

- 1 small pumpkin, halved, peeled, seeds removed, and pulp cubed
- 2 cups chicken broth
- 1 cup of coconut almond milk
- Sunflower seeds, pepper, thyme, and pepper, to taste

How To:

1. Add all the ingredients to a crockpot.
2. Close the lid.
3. Cook for 6-8 hours on LOW.
4. Make a smooth puree by employing a blender.
5. Garnish with roasted seeds.
6. Serve and enjoy!

Nutrition (Per Serving)

Calories: 60

Fat: 5g

Carbohydrates: 4g

Protein: 4g

Tomato Soup

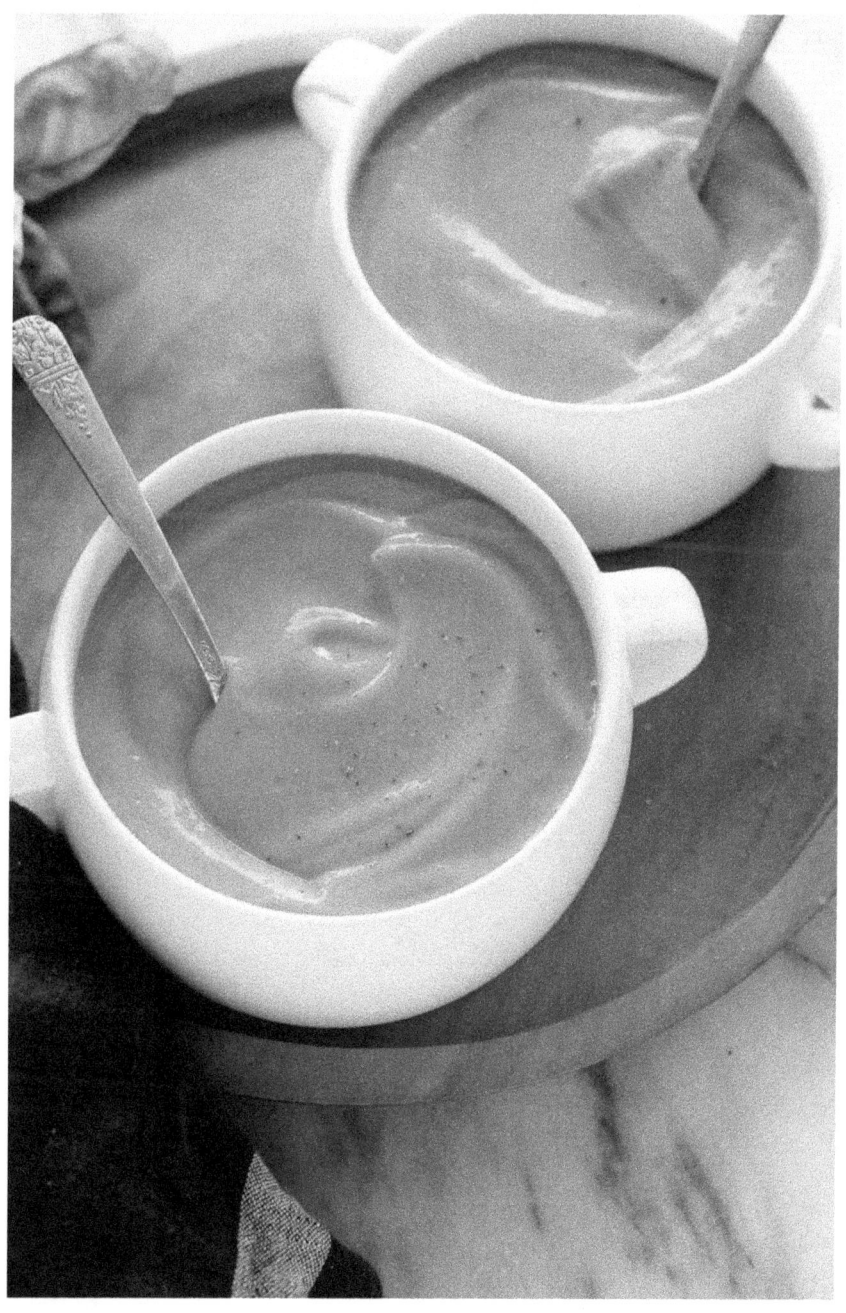

Serving: 3

Prep Time: 10 minutes

Cook Time: 6-8 hours

Ingredients:

- 4 cups water or vegetable broth
- 7 large tomatoes, ripe
- ½ cup macadamia nuts, raw
- 1 medium onion, chopped
- Sunflower seeds and pepper to taste

How To:

1. Take a nonstick skillet and add the onion.
2. Brown the onion for five minutes.
3. Add all the ingredients to a crockpot.
4. Cook for 6-8 hours on LOW.
5. Make a smooth puree by employing a blender.
6. Serve it warm and enjoy!

Nutrition (Per Serving)

Calories: 145

Fat: 12g

Carbohydrates: 8g

Protein: 6g

Pumpkin, Coconut and Sage Soup

Serving: 3

Prep Time: 10 minute

Cook Time: 30 minutes

Ingredients:

- 1 cup pumpkin, canned

- 6 cups chicken broth

- 1 cup low fat coconut almond milk

- 1 teaspoon sage, chopped

- 3 garlic cloves, peeled

- Sunflower seeds and pepper to taste

How To:

1. Take a stockpot and add all the ingredients except coconut almond milk into it.

2. Place stockpot over medium heat.
3. Let it bring back a boil.

4. Reduce heat to simmer for half-hour.
5. Add the coconut almond milk and stir.
6. Serve bacon and enjoy!

Nutrition (Per Serving)

Calories: 145

Fat: 12g

Carbohydrates: 8g

Protein: 6g

Sweet Potato and Leek Soup

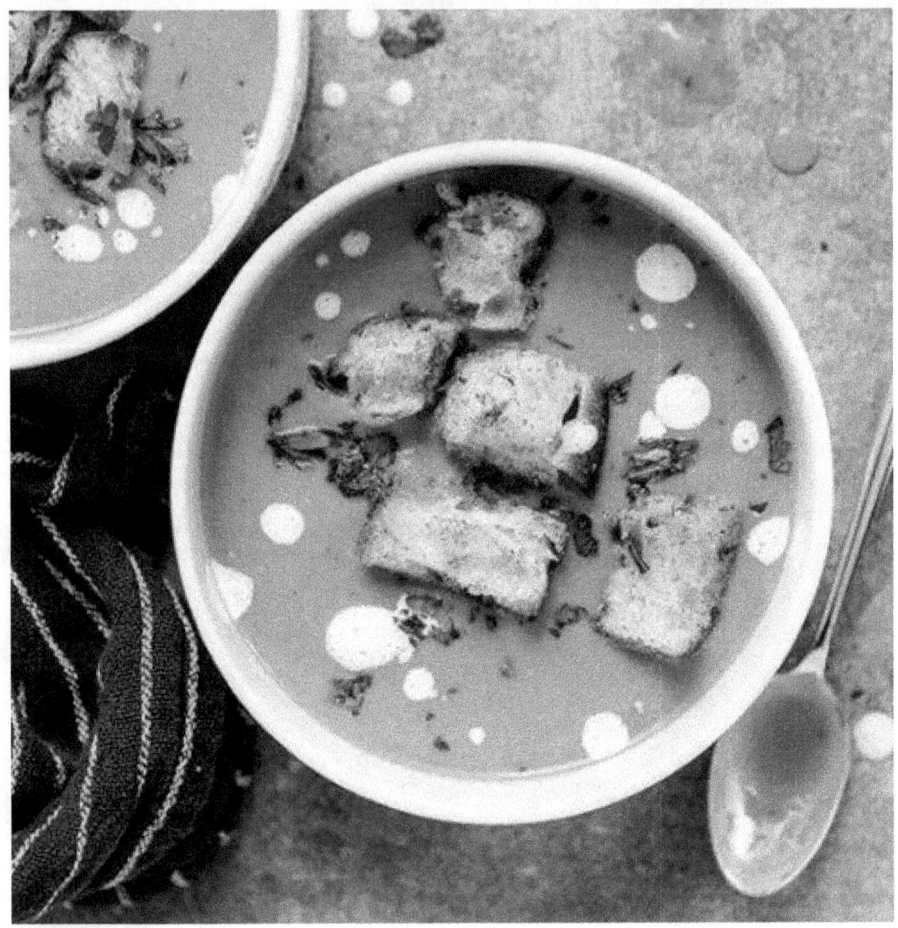

Serving: 6

Prep Time: 10 minutes

Cook Time: 8 hours

Ingredients:

- 6 cups sweet potatoes, peeled and cubed

- 2 leeks, whites and greens, sliced

- 6 cups vegetable stock

- 1 teaspoon dried thyme

- 1 teaspoon salt

- ¼ teaspoon fresh ground black pepper

How To:

1. Add sweet potatoes, leeks, thyme, stock, salt and pepper to your Slow Cooker.

2. Close lid and cook on LOW for 8 hours.
3. Mash with potato masher/ use an immersion blender to smooth the soup.
4. Serve and enjoy!

Nutrition (Per Serving)

Calories: 234

Fat: 2g
Carbohydrates: 47g

Protein: 8g

The Kale and Spinach Soup

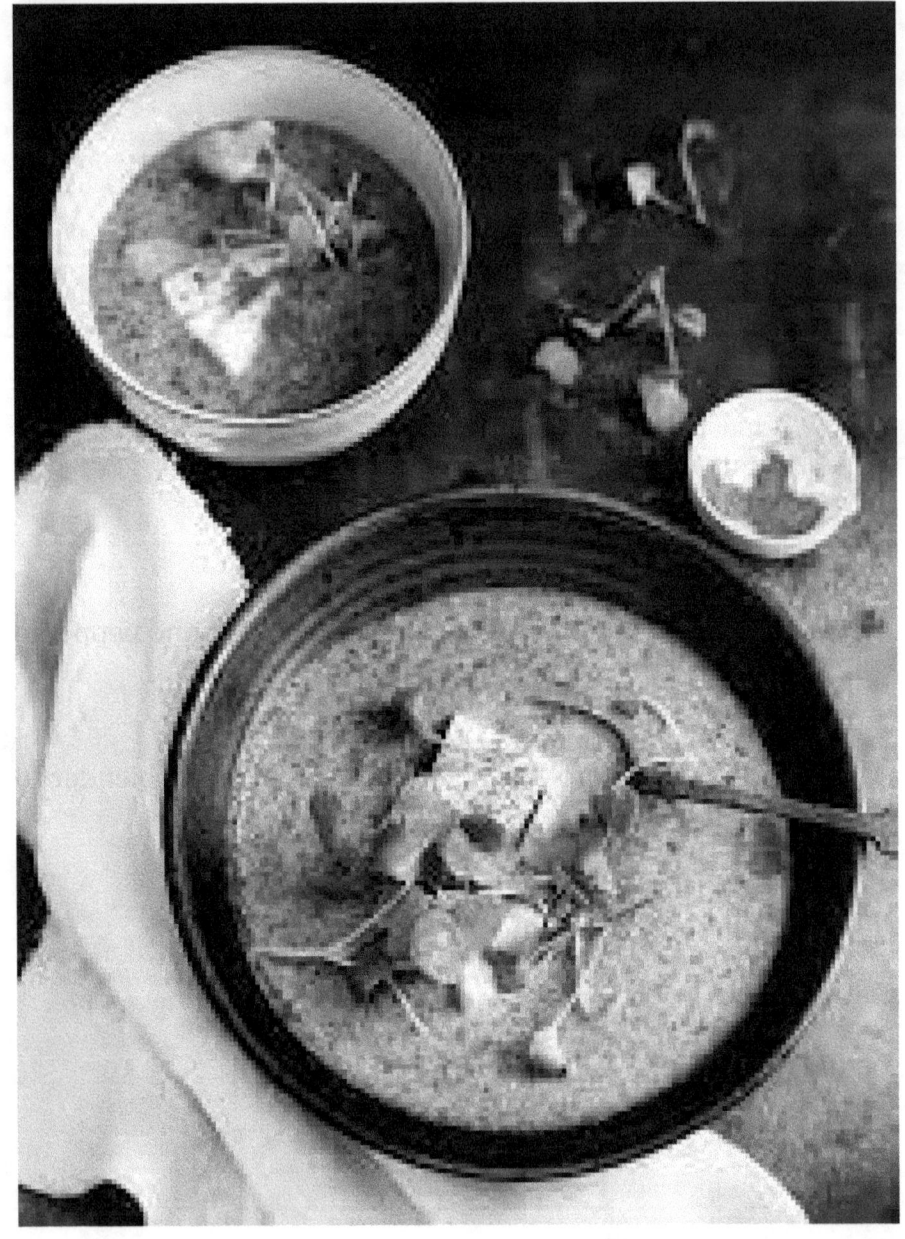

Serving: 4

Prep Time: 5 minutes

Cook Time: 10 minutes

Ingredients:

- 3 ounces coconut oil

- 8 ounces kale, chopped

- 2 avocados, diced

- 4 1/3 cups coconut almond milk

- Sunflower seeds and pepper to taste

How To:

1. Take a skillet and place it over medium heat. 2. Add kale and sauté for 2-3 minutes

2. Add kale to blender.

3. Add water, spices, coconut almond milk and avocado to blender also .
4. Blend until smooth and pour mix into bowl.
5. Serve and enjoy!

Nutrition (Per Serving)

Calories: 124

Fat: 13g

Carbohydrates: 7g

Protein: 4.2g

Japanese Onion Soup

Serving: 4

Prep Time: 15 minutes

Cook Time: 45 minutes

Ingredients:

- ½ stalk celery, diced

- 1 small onion, diced

- ½ carrot, diced

- 1 teaspoon fresh ginger root, grated

- ¼ teaspoon fresh garlic, minced

- 2 tablespoons chicken stock

- 3 teaspoons beef bouillon granules

- 1 cup fresh shiitake, mushrooms

- 2 quarts water

- 1 cup baby Portobello mushrooms, sliced

- 1 tablespoon fresh chives

How To:

1. Take a saucepan and place it over high heat, add water, bring back a boil.

2. Add beef bouillon, celery, onion, chicken broth , carrots, half the mushrooms, ginger, garlic.

3. placed on the lid and reduce heat to medium, cook for 45 minutes.

4. Take another saucepan and add another half mushroom.
5. Once the soup is cooked, strain the soup into the pot with uncooked mushrooms.
6. Garnish with chives and enjoy!

Nutrition (Per Serving)

Calories: 25

Fat: 0.2g

Carbohydrates: 5g

Protein: 1.4g

Amazing Broccoli and Cauliflower Soup

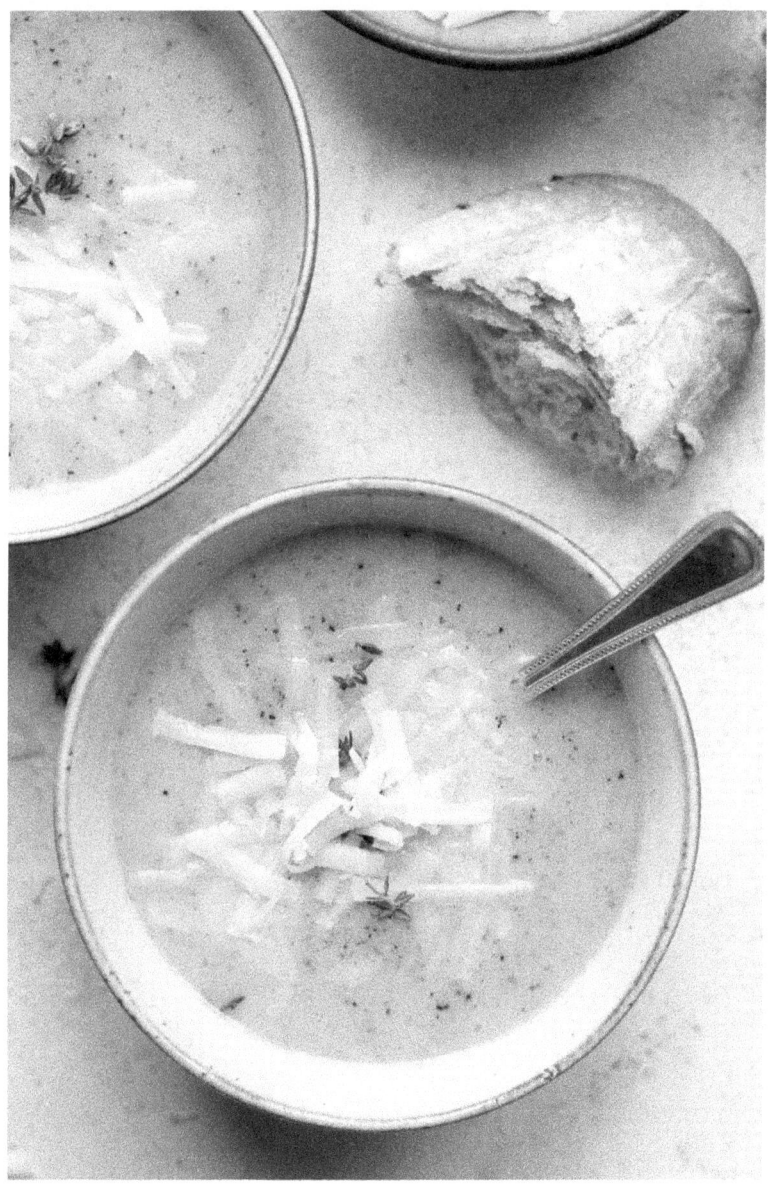

Serving: 4

Prep Time: 10 minutes

Cooking Time: 8 hours

Ingredients:

- 3 cups broccoli florets
- 2 cups cauliflower florets
- 2 garlic cloves, minced
- ½ cup shallots, chopped
- 1 carrot, chopped
- 3 ½ cups low sodium veggie stick
- Pinch of pepper
- 1 cup fat-free milk
- 6 ounces low-fat cheddar, shredded
- 1 cup non-fat Greek yogurt

How To:

1. Add broccoli, cauliflower, garlic, shallots, carrot, stock, pepper to your Slow Cooker.

2. Stir well and place lid.
3. Cook on LOW for 8 hours.
4. Add milk and cheese.

5. Use an immersion blender to smooth the soup.

6. Add yogurt and blend another time .
7. Ladle into bowls and enjoy!

Nutrition (Per Serving)

Calories: 218

Fat: 11g

Carbohydrates: 15g

Protein: 12g

Amazing Zucchini Soup

Serving: 4

Prep Time: 10 minutes

Cook Time: 20 minutes

Ingredients:

- 1 onion, chopped

- 3 zucchini, cut into medium chunks

- 2 tablespoons coconut milk

- 2 garlic cloves, minced

- 4 cups chicken stock

- 2 tablespoons coconut oil

- Pinch of salt

- Black pepper to taste

How To:

1. Take a pot and place over medium heat.
2. Add oil and let it heat up.
3. Add zucchini, garlic, onion and stir.
4. Cook for five minutes.
5. Add stock, salt, pepper and stir.
6. bring back a boil and reduce the warmth .
7. Simmer for 20 minutes.
8. Remove from heat and add coconut milk.
9. Use an immersion blender until smooth.
10. Ladle into soup bowls and serve.
11. Enjoy!

Nutrition (Per Serving)

Calories: 160

Fat: 2g

Carbohydrates: 4g

Protein: 7g

Portuguese Kale and Sausage Soup

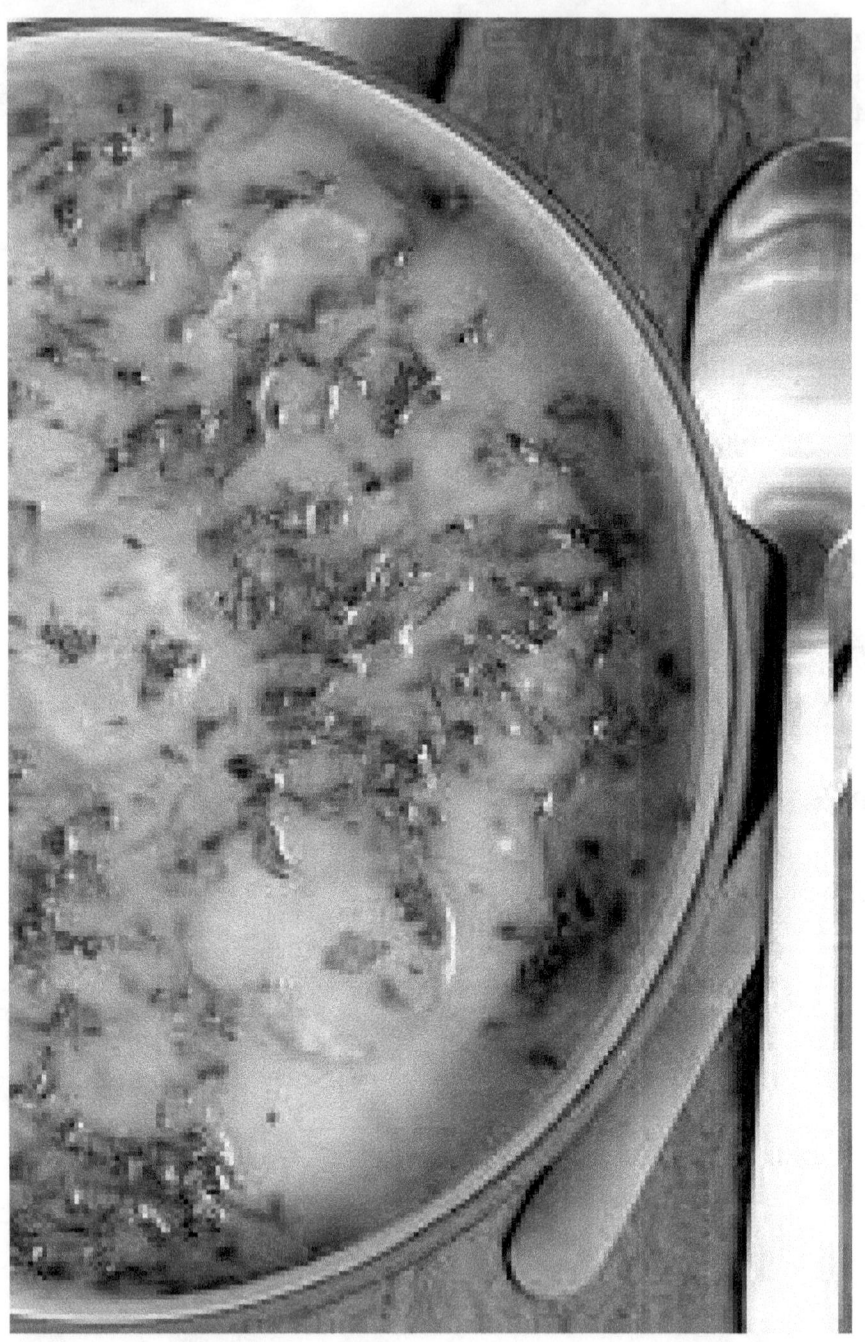

Serving: 4

Prep Time: 10 minutes

Cook Time: 35 minutes

Ingredients:

- 1 yellow onion, chopped

- 16 ounces sausage, chopped

- 3 sweet potatoes, chopped

- 4cups chicken stock1 pound kale, chopped pepper as needed

How To:

1. Take a pot and place it over medium heat.
2. Add sausage and brown each side .
3. Transfer to bowl.
4. Heat pot again over medium heat.
5. Add onion and stir for five minutes.
6. Add stock, sweet potatoes, stir and convey to a simmer.
7. Cook for 20 minutes.
8. Use an immersion blender to blend.
9. Add kale and pepper and simmer for two minutes over low heat.
10. Ladle soup to bowls and top with sausage with

pieces.
11.   Serve and enjoy!

Nutrition (Per Serving)

Calories: 200

Fat: 2g

Carbohydrates: 6g

Protein:8g

Dazzling Pizza Soup

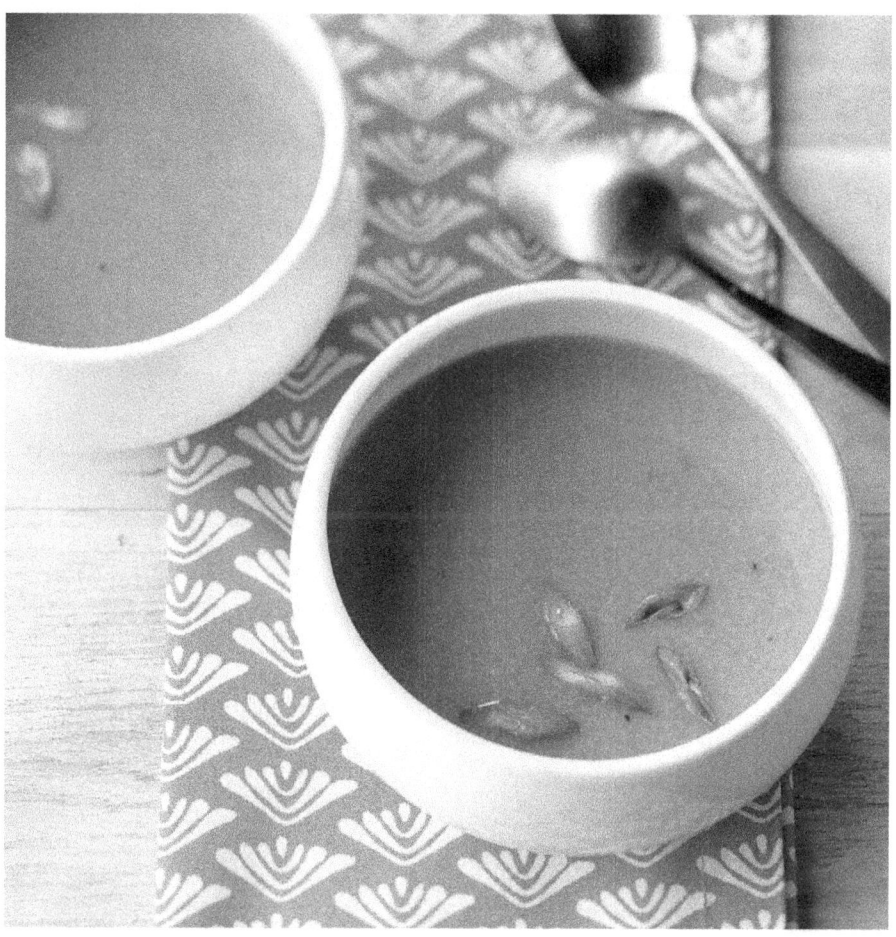

Serving: 6

Prep Time: 5 minutes

Cook Time: 30 minutes

Ingredients:

- 12 ounces chicken meat, sliced

- 4 ounces uncured pepperoni

- 1 can 25 ounces marinara

- 1 can 14.5 ounces fire roasted tomatoes

- 1 large onion, diced

- 15 ounces mushrooms, sliced

- 1 can 3 ounce sliced black olives

- tablespoon dried oregano

- 1 teaspoon garlic powder

- ½ teaspoon salt

How To:

1. Take large sized saucepan and add within the peperoni, chicken meat, marinara, onions, tomatoes, mushroom, oregano, olives, salt and garlic powder.
2. Cook the mixture for half-hour over medium level heat and soften the mushroom and onions.

3. Serve hot.

Nutrition (Per Serving)

Calories: 90

Fat: 2g

Carbohydrates: 17g

Protein: 3g

www.ingramcontent.com/pod-product-compliance
Lightning Source LLC
Chambersburg PA
CBHW070723030426
42336CB00013B/1903